T.I.H.
(TAP INTO HEALTH)
SIMPLE HEALTH AND HAPPINESS

Movin'
Melvin Brown

Content Selection, Arrangement, Co-editing * Francesca Sansalone

First editing * Jane Mackay

Photos * courtesy of Erick Regnard and other photographers

Cover Design and Interior Design * Alessio Luca Nuzzolo

MOVIN' MELVIN BROWN

TAP INTO HEALTH

T.I.H.: A LIFESTYLE SYSTEM FOR HEALTH AND HAPPINESS

THE BOOK ● SIMPLE HEALTH AND HAPPINESS

Gives you simple ways to change anything that doesn't work for you into things that do, and to get and stay healthy through food, exercise and thinking.

THE VIDEO ● LOW IMPACT HIGH OUTPUT WORKOUT SYSTEM

A low impact high output workout system suitable for about any age group, simple ways to get in shape and to stay that way.

THE DOUBLE CD ● MOTIVATIONAL RHYTHM TRACKS, INSPIRATIONAL SONGS

A doubled CD set of soul and gospel sounding rhythm tracks with inspirational, motivational lyrics especially written and designed for rhythm tap dancing with clap tracks to help you find and stay on the beat while you learn tap the easy way.

THE T-SHIRT ● IN MEMORY OF YOUR TRIP TO HEALTH AND HAPPINESS

In memory of where you are going and where you came from with Tap into Health.

www.movinmelvin.com

THE AUTHOR

Movin' Melvin Brown

THE MAN

Movin' Melvin is truly a Renaissance Man. He is a critically acclaimed singer, dancer, writer, philosopher and Man of Peace. His energy and his spirit light up any room, and he has devoted his life to sharing joy with the world.

Movin' Melvin has touched many hearts in Australia, Canada, Europe, Asia, Africa and the United States. His deep and cultivating laugh is so infectious that it can make audiences forget about their worries and live for that moment of happiness. He is an absorbing storyteller and shares his incisive philosophy with his audience. His shows inspire and entertain worldwide audiences through song, dance, storytelling and humor.

A lifetime of entertaining on stage, television and film, as well as his numerous recordings and writings, has led to the creation of his Musicals "A Man, A Magic, A Music", which has received awards and five star reviews in major International Arts Festivals around the world; 'Me, Ray Charles and Sammy Davis Jr', 'Soul to Soul (I Have a Dream)' and 'The Ray Charles Experience'.

What a refreshing sense of hope this man brings to the world...

THE SONG AND DANCE MAN

Imagine a voice that embraces all styles of music, each with as much feeling as the other. That is the voice of *Movin'* Melvin Brown. His sound has been compared to such great entertainers as Otis Redding, Ray Charles, James Brown, Sam Cooke, Louis Armstrong, Sammy Davis Jr, and many of the gospel greats.

His intriguing shows have entertained all age groups at major International Arts Festivals, among which include Edinburgh, Avignon, Sydney, Vancouver, and Orlando; as well as Las Vegas Show Lounges, MGM Grand, Jupiter's Casino in Australia, gospel shows and other worldwide events. He has performed on the "World art Stage"/BBC at The Edinburgh Festival, and he was the only act to be called back for three different shows because of popular demand by the audience.

Movin' Melvin has been called "the man with the fastest moving dance feet". He has combined the styles of many of the masters including Fred Astaire, Sammy Davis Jr, Bojangles, Gene Kelly, Gregory Hines and The Nicholas Brothers to create his high energy shows. His dancing talents include Tap Dancing, Juke Dancing, Clogging, Jazz, Swing, Contemporary, and Robotics. Audiences enjoy watching his dance moves that reflect styles from the 1940's into the new millennium. *Movin'* Melvin is truly The Last of the Great Song and Dance Men!

The media love him! *Movin'* Melvin has appeared on major TV shows in all of the countries where he has performed, including CNN International from The Art Deco Festival in Miami, BBC coverage on the Edinburgh Festival, GMA, In Melbourne Tonight, and Club Buggery Sydney, RAI Rome, RTE Madrid, France2, etc. He has also appeared in a number of films including The Minstrel Man, Home by Midnight, The Red Headed Stranger, A Pair of Aces and

Another Pair of Aces with Willie Nelson. He was also featured tap dancing to Mozart's music in a Sydney Australia Tourism commercial!

THE "I LOVE YOU DAY" PROJECT

Melvin travels the world with the message that "Love is the answer to our problems". He believes that everything that exists began with a thought, and so he promotes the idea that we start everything with the Thought of Love.

To promote this philosophy, Melvin established February 2 as "I Love You Day". On this very special day he has performed concerts filled with love songs he has written to help bring the world together for a positive event based on thought of love. Melvin began promoting "I Love You Day" to the world on February 2, 2001, with the first I Love You Day concert held on February 2, 2002, in Sydney. He continues to promote this project each year with concerts in various international locations.

Melvin sums up his reasons for establishing "I Love You Day" as follows, "When I change, the world will change, and the world will love when I love." For project updates check out www.ILoveYouDay.com.

THE "CHANGE THIS WORLD" PROJECT

Movin' Melvin made a commitment to change the world many years ago when he started the "Change This World" project in Austin, Texas. He believes that to change the world and make it a better place for all of us to live, we must start with the children. We must teach children to love and to understand each other.

Melvin's dream of building a home for homeless children and elderly people has begun to come true, thanks to all the support he has received around the world. He is supporting his project with his entertainment income, and through the sale of his Videos -Tap Dance into Health, The Best of *Movin'* Melvin, as well as his several CDs. Melvin has written a special song entitled **"Change This World"**, in support of this project, and the sales of his books also provide financial support for this project.

Thanks to everyone who is helping to Change this World!

For the latest news visit *www.movinmelvin.com*

INTRODUCTION

The Mission

I am here for a purpose, to become the person that I want to see, and to create that world that I want to live in. By becoming the person that I want to see I then have a means to offer to others around me to become the person that they want to see and be.

The world around me will never change unless I do so first, then the world I live in has no choice but to change, and it is the same for everyone else, this is my simple message to all.

It is through unconsciousness that we have fallen into a place of unbalance where on one side we have all of the necessary resources for health and happiness but suffer from malnutrition, obesity, sickness, and disease, while on the other side we have people dying from hunger every ten seconds, children suffering from malnutrition, and the same sickness and disease as we see from the side where the people have more than the means to eliminate this from their lives and the lives of others.

Through TIH we can do this.

This is the balance that we seek which is very simple, a back to the basics approach for everyone, this means taking the best from and for your life and leaving the rest, this is the purpose of TIH to help those who have the means to use them in a way that they eliminate malnutrition, obesity, sickness and disease, and through their thinking come to health and happiness, then take the resources (money) from the sale of my TIH system and supply those on the other side with the same benefits so as to bring everyone to the center to a place of health and happiness.

TIH is a way to make a complete difference for everyone.

MANY THANKS to everyone who has been inspiring me to keep looking for more answers: my children, my manager, my family, my friends and wonderful audiences around the world and most of all God for the opportunity to serve.

THE BOOK STATEMENT

This is all about your life of health and happiness. Although you may begin to see changes overnight or right away, the system is designed to bring you to a point of health and happiness (for life) over a reasonable period of time by implementing small, simple things into your life at a non-stressful level, taking you to the point where you wake up feeling, thinking, and being on top of the world with no need to look back.

This is your Life. Just do it.

SIMPLE SECRETS TO HEALTH AND HAPPINESS

The secret to health and happiness is your thinking. In order to feel good things, to see good things, and to do good things, you must first think good things. Look around you at what you have in and around your life, and then ask yourself, "Where and when in my life did I give emotional thought (positive or negative) to these situations that I now have," and you will have found the source of your situation as it is today. Bad or good thoughts create equally bad or good results; the only variable is how much you think about either, and that can be readily seen by the way you feel right now. Simply put, when you feel good you look good; when you look good, you act good; when you act good, you do good; and when you do good, you feel good—it makes a circle leading back to your original thought.

In life it's as simple as seeing the glass as half full or half empty, God has given you freedom of choice, and with it the power to choose good or bad, full or empty; everything in and around you is working off of that choice that you make.

Your weight, your job, your relationship—your everything that you do is coming through your head or your thinking. God makes that choice available to everyone equally.

Let's look at the most emotional situations for most: death. You could think that God or the universe, which has infinite intelligence, has death planned into it, or simply that the person made a choice to leave, or that they have served their purpose and have made a choice to move on up the ladder to a higher place. This kind of thinking would allow you to celebrate the time they gave to you by coming here, and then you can feel happy about their going on to where they need to go.

Or you could think that it is a dark dreadful ending to a life at its end and feel unhappy.

Now you can see that it simply the way you look at the situation that determines how you feel, because it is your thinking that is the source of your happiness or unhappiness.

Listen to your thoughts. I mean, really pay attention to what you think when you are thinking it. When you do this you can readily see that you have the power to change it, as with anything else in your life, to what you want it to be.

Give your thinking only to that which serves you and your health and happiness, and in the process you will serve God and all around you from that which you have.

THE PLACE WHERE YOU TAKE

CONTROL OF YOUR THINKING IS THE

SAME PLACE WHERE YOU TAKE

CONTROL OF YOUR LIFE

SIMPLE LIFE

The reason that you are reading this material is that you have made a decision to be healthy and happy, and what you are doing now is getting information to get there and remain that way.

Knowledge is power, the power you need to change, and self-knowledge is the power to change yourself.

We live in a time of addiction, to food, alcohol, money, drugs, and so on. The simple truth is that to change anything, you must first give yourself a good enough reason to change. This is the only real means of changing something towards health and happiness.

Many people have tried to change something like dieting, or smoking, or learning a new language, only to find themselves back at the start again and again.

I remember a story with my ex-wife. She was trying to quit smoking and lose weight. After a couple of years of trying, she was ready to give up, complaining that it was too hard to change and she just couldn't do it.

At this point I explained that you can do anything, but you simply have to give yourself a good enough reason to do it. She replied, "I can't do it." I replied, "You can, you just haven't given yourself a good enough reason to change, because anyone can change if they give themselves a good enough reason to." She replied, "I have, but it didn't work." I replied, "The reason wasn't good enough." I then asked her, "Do you love your children?" She said, "Yes." I then asked, "If someone came along with a gun and put it to your kids' heads and told you that if you ever smoke another cigarette they would pull the trigger, would you stop smoking then?" She replied, "Of course I would." I then said, "You would stop smoking because you have a good enough reason to."

This is true of human beings. We change if we can give ourselves a good enough reason to change. This involves first of all a decision, and then a purpose, which is a reason—a good enough reason. A reason that you have taken time to think about and even gather information on so as to fully convince yourself that you want to change. With that, you have the basis for real, permanent change. This is true of anything and everything in your life.

Health and happiness (life) must be important to you, important enough to you to be willing to think about it and make decisions about your life every step of the way, so as to make sure that you have the best that this life has to offer. This is what you deserve, and only you can give it to you, by changing those things in your life that don't work for you into things that do work for you.

So basically speaking, the real way to change is reason.

SIMPLE REASON

The reason for TIH is to allow you to build a body and mind that you can live with in health and happiness for the rest of your life.

The body is God's temple, and every religion or spiritual teaching advocates that it is a source that we must recognize, show appreciation to, that we must give thanks to for the opportunity and chance to have and celebrate consciously here.

There are many names and titles used to describe the source of our existence, because when you can find and give yourself a source, for the good of your existence, you can walk forward on a firm foundation that allows you to see the bad, and then put it behind you in view of that good. This allows us to live, see, and appreciate the good or the beauty of it all, on a conscious and free level. I choose to use the word God, but no matter what name you use or don't use, in the end it all must go back to the source.

No matter what we are and have accomplished in our lives, there is one thing that stands in front of it all: reason. All of what we did not accomplish had the same source, but from the other end. What I am saying is that you have to give yourself a good enough reason to do anything, no matter what it is, or you are not likely to do it. The truth of this is simple to find. Just look at your life and what you have achieved and what you haven't—you will find reason as the bottom line.

Man is a rational being in the sense that he has the faculties to think and reason. If we don't think (or sometimes allow others to do it for us), then we don't reason and we don't rationalize properly, so we keep waking up to a life that feels like someone else or something else is choosing for us, because we know that we would not choose that (consciously). So when we neglect two of our greatest assets, the ability to think and to reason, we can easily stand seemingly alone and lost from the source of our existence. The best part of this is that as long as we are alive here we have the opportunity to find God or to find a good reason for our existence to live by, to, or with through our own reasoning.

Today, all you have to do is to balance yourself and live, and if you find yourself in tomorrow, then the balance of now is also the past, the present, and future of your life.

The work of your being is to be. And to be here in balance you must have a foundation to balance on. This is the first and last source of love, health, and happiness.

IT IS MY BELIEF

THAT SICKNESS AND DISEASE

ARE FIRST HELD IN PLACE BY WHAT

YOU BELIEVE OR DON'T BELIEVE,

AND CAN BE TRACED BACK TO WHAT

YOU EAT OR DON'T EAT.

TEN SIMPLE STEPS TO HEALTH AND HAPPINESS

The Beginning

The first thing that you should understand is that you do not have to be at war with yourself to find health and happiness.

Because what you are currently doing is what you decided on at some point in time with the idea of bringing about health and happiness, and what you decided on is likely habit now. You now realize that health and happiness are only partially or not at all recognized in your life, but you now have them in habit form and they seem to be repeating themselves in your life, while you still continue your search for health and happiness.

The truth is, though it's said that it's hard to break a habit, habits can be easily broken instantly, but most people don't do that until they are put in a situation where they think they have no other choice, such as a life-threatening disease, death of a loved one, trauma or great rewards, and so on, otherwise the habit stays there doing its thing on you.

This is another simple and reasonable approach to changing those habits that do not serve your life, or your purpose in life. That way is TIH. This system is based on small and simple modifications of what you are already doing, which make big and lasting changes in your life.

The TIH plan is a life plan for health and happiness. This is a physical, mental, and practical system, to get you to health and happiness with your whole life from this point on by simple, easy, and practical means. It's so simple—you use what you have to get what you want, and to take the work out of it. It's more like acquiring a taste for something little by little until you become so attuned to it that at some point it does its work on you without your having to stop and think about it anymore—it's just happening.

The habit of true health and happiness is God's plan for you. Now make it your plan for you.

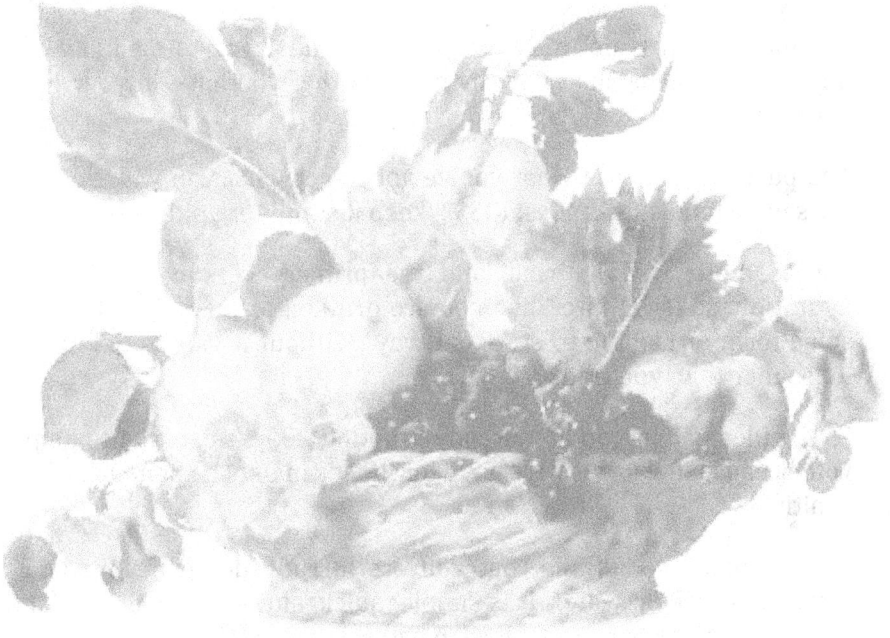

"LET FOOD BE THY MEDICINE AND

MEDICINE BE THY FOOD"

Hippocrates

STEP ONE

The idea of TIH is not to stress you or to cause you to mentally or physically work against ingrained habits that you have in your life and system.

The purpose is to use what you've got to get what you want, or as the saying in business goes: KISS ("keep it simple, stupid").

For example, we all drink, and the primary reason for this is hydration, so if you are alive you are drinking or taking in fluid in some form or fashion to stay that way (without it you would die a lot sooner than you think).

So the idea is that you are already drinking, so let's use that to help you, because if water is necessary for life it can only be beneficial for health.

So let's make something that you are already doing benefit you more, by drinking water. It is simple, quick, and very beneficial for you and your system, and it has no bad side effects.

Not only does water keep you alive, but it also keeps you healthy by flushing toxins out of your system. It helps the blood to flow and oxidize better, which helps the heart, the brain, and all of your vital organs.

Simple plain old water, H_2O. It's simple, available and it composes a large majority of your body weight, so it's really important.

I drink it, you drink it, and everybody drinks it. Why? Because it's vital to life, and with just a simple little modification it can make a great difference to you and your system.

This is how we do it.

Most people wake up somewhat dehydrated in the morning, because even when you sleep your body has to keep doing its work to keep you alive. Work is the use of energy, and any time you use energy you lose water, or burn it from your system. So this is what we want to do. When you get up in the morning keep on doing whatever you usually do, but first have a glass of water before you do it. If it is coffee, if it is tea, a smoothie, breakfast, whatever it is you do first thing in the morning, just drink a glass of water first.

Now if you are the kind of person who needs to have an in-between meal snack, it's OK, just have a glass of water before that too, then have your snack.

Then before lunch—yes, again, have a glass of water fifteen minutes to a half hour before lunch. The time is only important if you have it; if you forget or for some reason you don't or can't have the water fifteen minutes to a half hour before lunch, just do it while you wait for your food or prepare your food. Just do it before, that's the important thing.

If you have an afternoon snack or beverage, drink the water before that. And then before dinner—yes, you guessed it, have a glass of water fifteen minutes to a half hour before dinner.

This will yield big benefits. Quite often when people are thirsty they think that they are hungry, so they eat. If they would simply drink first they would know afterwards if they are really hungry and want to eat. If you are overweight you will lose pounds, because you will eat less as a result of drinking the water, and you will find that your system will be better regulated as you start to flush out more toxins. In just a short time you will notice that you feel better. These are all worth the price of a glass of water.

This will become habit after a short time, and it is a habit that you can live with the rest of your life. Water is the real low-calorie, high-energy inexpensive diet drink, for health and happiness, so for the next thirty days (this is how long it takes to form a habit), get the water into your system. Don't worry about the other stuff you may or may not be doing. Just start with this and continue until it's time for step two.

Each step is a thirty-day, one-step-at-a-time plan, so focus on this and do it for thirty days, and then move on to the next step.

STEP TWO

On average most people have salad at some point during their meal. If not, chances are that you are not getting enough vitamins in your diet (most people who do not eat salad usually don't have other raw fruits and vegetables either), which means that you like a lot of people in developed countries suffer from malnutrition. This simply means that you don't get the proper amount of nutrients from your diet to stay balanced, or to maintain a normal standard of health where you feel good, look good, and function good from what you eat.

I think that at least half of what you eat during the day should be fresh vegetables.

Again, this is a simple modification to what you are doing when you sit down to eat your salad first. But if you are not eating live fruits and vegetables (this means fruits and vegetables in their natural state that have not been cooked or processed), it is likely that you are malnourished.

So if you are eating salad make it a habit to eat it first. If you are not eating salad, start to implement it little by little into you eating routine. Salad can be anything from a full range of countless fruits and vegetables. It is likely that if you start to try then you will find something that you really like, and if you make a habit of looking for what you like, you will find more of it, because we find what look for in life in all ways.

But again, make this simple adjustment: first eat your salad or whatever vegetable that you can get, and then eat whatever else you have been eating. If it is fruit, try to eat it at least ten minutes before.

What you accomplish: 1) You get your nutrition first (that is the first reason that you eat), so you have already satisfied your body's need for nutrition. 2) You will not be as hungry and you will not eat as much of anything else that will distract from your health and well-being.

The fact is that God and the universe provide what we need to eat in the form we need it ready to eat. We as mankind have tried to prove that we know better by cooking or modifying or processing the food. You only need look around to see the unhealthiness, sickness, and disease in our society to understand that what man has really proved is his incompetence. As a result, each of us must take responsibility for our life and the source (food being one), so that we can get the maximum benefit from what we eat. Keep in mind it can be good and good for you at the same time, so you don't have to give up anything—you are actually getting something new.

So the simple modification is to eat your salad or fresh veggies first.

Each step is a thirty-day, one-step-at-a-time plan, so focus on this and do it for thirty days, and then move on to the next step.

STEP THREE

The old saying that "an apple a day keeps the doctor away" is more than just an old saying—it has a lot of real truth in it: most fruits have a load of vitamins in them, including, of real importance, vitamin C.

Sure there are a lot of supplements and synthetic things on the market that are supposed to replace or replenish the vitamins in your system, but I believe—and it has been proven time and time again—that man is no match for nature.

In spite of all that we have done to compete, with the development of food processing, canning, and other methods, the best source for nutrients is nature. So whether it's an apple from a tree, a berry from a vine, or any other fruit, the very best place to get it is from the place it grows; the next best place is from someone who has done that for you, a farmers market or grocery store, or where you can find it, but try to get it from as close to the source as possible. You may need to wash the fruit, but you are still much better off with the real thing: fresh fruit from the tree or the vine.

There are those of the school of thought that sugar is not necessarily good for you, but there is a place where what nature provides and what man makes have to be separated. Unfortunately, what man makes in the way of sugar serves more his pocket than your health, and if the motivation is wrong then the product is likely the same. Mother Nature on the other hand has pure and simple motivation: life (or the implementation of life and growth), and it has no match, so what you get from fresh fruit is the pure sweetness of nature with its only motivation to serve you and your health, so it has to be good for you.

Now the case for fresh fruit has been made, this is the next small and simple implementation to add to your life. First take a look at the large range of fruits and vegetables that are available to you, then sort through them by eating to see what you really like, then in between meals just eat one piece before you eat what you may usually eat in between meals. The idea is to have at least two pieces of fruit a day. If you make it a habit to eat fruit at snack time before you have anything else, it will be something easier to start and keep doing. The best thing about this is you will notice that you are not getting sick or bothered with seasonal illness as much.

So in between meals whatever you have been doing you don't have to stop, just start eating a piece of fruit before it.

Each step is a thirty-day, one-step-at-a-time plan, so focus on this and do it for thirty days, and then move on to the next step.

STEP FOUR

SIMPLE NUTRITION

We live in a world where every three-point-six seconds a person dies from starvation (so in the time that it takes entertain a single thought, one life passes). I have just read the statistics that in this world in which we live, one-third of the people are dying from starvation, one-third are malnourished, and one-third live in abundance, and a big percentage of them suffer from malnutrition (which means that they have the opportunity to eat the right food for nutrition, but are taking in more non-food than food).

In spite of these statistics, there is enough food to feed everyone with nutritional adequacy; we just have to come to understand the concept of sharing and caring for all of life as we wish to have it.

Nutrition is nourishment for your body, or a level of vitamins and minerals that will allow your body to sustain and attain life.

This simply means that what you eat and drink should have nutrients in it to be considered food or nourishment; if it doesn't then it's simply not considered food. Your health and your happiness are your responsibility, and no one or nothing can or will take those away from you.

Yes, we have government agencies and other people who should and would serve our basic interests, especially when it comes to the vitals of life like food and water, but quite often (more and more), these two essentials are not given priority, so the information may be available, but unless you are really looking for it you may not get it. This can readily be seen in all of the non-food marketing that we are constantly being subjected to.

I have advocated for a long time that the number one job of the government should be to educate the people so they can have the power to make decisions about their lives, especially in the area of vitals like food and drink. People do not make the right decisions because they do not have the knowledge to do so. When you look around at the amount of overweight, unhealthy and sick people in our society we can clearly see that people are in need of education about to live healthily.

For a very simple example, let's say that you pay twenty million dollars to have a house built (you are buying the top of the line)—your expectation should be that this house will last for a lifetime, and that it serve well your needs for protection, comfort and shelter, without your having to constantly put money into it (you only need to do what's necessary to maintain the level that you have) to fix or repair it.

This is exactly what your body is about. You come into this life with the perfect body (to all intents and purposes). Where we have lost most of the time is through a lack of education about our life and our body—so this is the vital step you should take now.

Look, look, and look; read, read and read the labels on what you buy to consume. Get a natural nutrition book and learn about what you are reading on the labels, even if you only read a page a day; after all, you have time, it's your life we are talking about, so get the information so you can live in health and happiness.

Read and understand nutrients: where they are and what they do. It's a small step with big results.

Each step is a thirty-day, one-step-at-a-time plan, so focus on this and do it for thirty days, and then move on to the next step.

STEP FIVE

SIMPLE SWEET

The saying is "it's not so much what you are eating, as it is what's eating you." Living in America I am able to see directly the results of what overeating and undernourishment mean. The last century has seen a rapid rise in lifestyle diseases, such as diabetics, obesity, cancer, and other associated illnesses that now plague us as a society. Not only do we eat too much, but we eat too much of the wrong things, and that is where the real problem comes in. First we should understand that lifestyle diseases are those that come from the habits that harm our minds and our bodies, and at the top of this ladder is our food and drink. This is something that you definitely have control over, so actually you can say that sickness and disease is something that you choose by not taking advantage of the right things.

What are those right things? They are the things that Mother Nature gives us for food and it is still in its natural state—this is as possible as it is not.

In a sense we are being processed to death. What that means is that food manufactures as a rule strip all of the nutrients out of the food that they put in the stores and leave you with addictive substances to help you destroy your system with.

I need to say in their defense that by the time we get what we consider to be food to eat, even the people who are selling it have no idea of what's in it or what it actually does to you.

We live in a country where the pharmaceutical and the medical industries are two of the biggest industries in the country, and they are armed with the knowledge that if you ingest all of the processed so-called food stuff that is put into the stores, you have no choice but to get sick. And then they condition you to believe that they have the ways and means to heal you, which is just another part of a bad puzzle, because there is only one who can heal you and Jesus spoke of that being when he said, "You are healed by your faith."

The only thing that should and will supersede this is that an "ounce of prevention is worth a pound of cure." Simply put, if you eat what's good for you to begin with, you will likely not need to be cured of any sickness.

I hope that I have painted a bad enough scenario for what I am suggesting for your next step—removing white refined sugar from your diet. This product has been called deadly, and for all of the real damage it does to your body I am inclined to agree. So the next step is to again read—to know all of the names they put on the labels that are really just refined sugar, then eliminate it from your life, while you still have a life, and replace it with raw unprocessed sweets such as honey and plant-derived sweeteners. Whatever you use, make sure it is natural (and unprocessed), and use it in moderation.

In a very short time you will notice a difference in how you feel and function, so take the step.

Each step is a thirty-day, one-step-at-a-time plan, so focus on this and do it for thirty days, and then move on to the next step.

STEP SIX

SIMPLE HEALTH AND HAPPINESS

The idea of happiness is not to look at or for the things that make you unhappy, because whatever you put your attention on grows and gets bigger in your life, and what you take your attention away from gets smaller and goes away from your life.

When we speak of white processed flour, we are really talking about something that leads to strokes, heart attacks, high blood pressure—just to name a few of the things that can be the end result of ingesting this substance.

Whereas whole grains (wheat or unprocessed flour) and natural flour from other sources like rice, almonds and other alternatives that can be used to replace white processed flour are things that (as opposed to just look and taste) actually have nutrients, and are healthy in reasonable amounts.

Our attention should be on those things that serve us and give us life, and you should know that there are natural alternatives to anything that you get on the market that is unhealthy for you to consume; it just takes a little effort and time, but this will serve you well in the end.

So your attention should be on what you want to become and on being healthy and happy. Stay conscious of that and the more you look the more you will find. Then you will realize at some point that you have a choice, and it is now you who is making that choice.

Remember that knowledge is power, the power to change, so the more you look for healthy and wholesome things to eat, the more you will find them, thus allowing you to freely connect with your goal for health and happiness.

The main thing to remember is that in the end it doesn't cost more to eat healthily. If you eat truly nutritional food, first of all you are likely to eat less, because your body will no longer give you a hunger signal because it has the nutrients it needs to do its work. And in the end you will spend less money, because you are not consuming as much, and you spend less time being sick and paying for doctor visits and losing time from work. So in the end, eating healthy will cost less and give more to your life.

So step three is to find and use healthy alternatives to white processed flour, and incorporate them into your eating. Find the alternatives and begin to put them in place of the unhealthy and allow this practice to become habit.

Each step is a thirty-day, one-step-at-a-time plan, so focus on this and do it for thirty days, and then move on to the next step.

STEP SEVEN

SIMPLE TASTE

We live in a society that is pretty much addicted to taste, and regrettably not to the taste of food itself (which would be great in this sense), but to what we put on and in or cook into the food we eat, so much so that what we sit down to eat we don't have an idea of what it really tastes like.

This is so because the food industry has done a real job of getting and keeping us addicted to what they put into the food. One main source of that addiction is salt, preservatives, monosodium, sodium, and all of the other masked or unmasked names that they give to salt that often keep you unaware of what it actually is.

The fact is that most people would actually laugh if they actually knew the things that salt is put into, often for no apparent reason, and it makes no sense except to keep you hooked on it.

What I am speaking of is what we call normal table salt, which is only a chemical with no nutrients whatsoever.

This chemical has been linked to heart disease, strokes, high blood pressure, headaches, and obesity, just to name a few, so the question is why does the food industry want to keep you addicted to this chemical? Because when you are addicted to salt most everything that you eat will only taste of salt, so when you don't taste that in or with your food you think that the food has no taste, so they can keep selling you all of the non-food that they want to no matter how its packaged; your addiction tells you that it's good. The food manufacturers can and will put anything on the shelf in the store in a great-looking jar, can or box, and you unknowingly buy it as food—they can make money and you get little more than health problems for the money that you spend.

As I said they have many names for the same ingredient, salt, so when you go to read the label first understand what it is you are reading. The next step is to read up on the problems that salt can bring to you, and then when you fully understand, look for an alternative, things like kelp, seaweed granules, even just dried sea salt has nutritional content, or there are a whole host of herbs out there that you can flavor your food with and get some real nutrients in the process. Use any of these things for flavor to a small extent and little by little you will discover the real taste of what you eat—and that's the point (outside of nutrients) of eating it.

It's all so simple ... if you are going to eat for taste, at least taste what you are eating.

Each step is a thirty-day, one-step-at-a-time plan, so focus on this and do it for thirty days, and then move on to the next step.

STEP EIGHT

SIMPLE VITAMINS

America is probably one of the most overfed and undernourished countries in the world. What I am talking about are real vitamins and minerals.

How sick you get, how long you stay sick, the disease you contract, how much you suffer, and how you age and die can all be directly connected to what you consume.

The basic fact is after your thoughts, what you eat and drink are the next most important factors in your life.

So to eliminate these lower equations, we need to seek proper nutrition and use it as a part of our everyday life, just like walking and talking. In order for us to get anything or something we must first be able to recognize it, and where we are today, many of us don't even recognize it.

God and the universe has provided us with everything we could need for health and revitalization of our body in the form that is best used by us, but we have decided that we know better than nature, even if we can plainly see that we could never hope to duplicate what nature does.

We take what comes from the perfect source, such as fruits, vegetables, and grains, and attempt to make it better by cooking or processing it and as a result we wind up with mostly garbage. Or as is the case in so called first-world countries, we end up with pretty garbage, with little or no nutritional content.

There is a simple rule for happiness: find and choose that which adds to your life in the best ways, and leave the rest behind.

It is the same with food. Find the food you like (in its natural state with all of its nutrients intact), eat it, and leave the rest behind you. And don't look back.

If you want the best of anything in life, you go directly to the source.

Slight modification can be good such as with Japanese food, which is usually just braised on the outside with very high heat, so that there are still nutrients intact inside the food.

Eating for health and happiness is really very simple, the closer you are to the source with fruits and vegetables, the more nutrients you get from it. For instance, if you pick an apple from a tree, rinse it, and eat it, you get the maximum amount of nutrients it has to offer.

So if you are overweight, underweight, sickly, diseased, or just wanting to look and feel better, you will likely find the problem and the solution in what you are thinking, eating, or drinking; that's all there is.

Step eight is when you sit down to eat, first take time to look at what you are about to eat, and simply ask yourself: Where are my nutrients? If you can't readily see where your vitamins or minerals are coming from, then it's time for you to decide either to keep doing what you are doing, and getting what you are getting, or to start at that moment to get what you need to get what you want: health and happiness. It's your decision.

Each step is a thirty-day, one-step-at-a-time plan, so focus on this and do it for thirty days, and then move on to the next step.

STEP NINE

If you are to reach the point of health and happiness, you must first answer and understand one question: Why do I eat and drink?

The simple and logical answer is to replenish and restore the nutrients and fluids that your body is constantly using up or secreting.

If you don't eat and drink, you don't live, so basically everything that you put into your mouth to eat is either adding to or taking away from your health, and thus your happiness.

The human body is amazing, as it will continue to function for a long time on very few vitamins, but then after so long it starts to lose its ability to keep healthy, which shows up in the form of sickness, disease, pain, other physical disorders, and even life-threatening illness. I have noticed that between the ages of forty to fifty-five is when sickness or major illness shows up in most people's life, and it is because they have been depriving their body of vitamins for too long and now it's starting to let them know in a big way.

Basically, the will to live must be accompanied by the will to eat and to drink properly so that that happens.

A simple way to understand this is to think of it like pouring dirty water through a filter—if you constantly do this then the filter will get more and more clogged until eventually no water can flow through it. So now one of two things will happen: the filter will not allow anything to flow through, or it will break, and you will have the same result.

This is in effect what happens to your body when you fail to put nutrients in it. So step nine is whenever you sit down to eat, first take a few seconds to relax and be present, and then look at what you are about to eat and ask yourself: Where are my vitamins? Keep asking yourself this question until you actually become aware of what you are putting into your mouth.

Again, knowledge is power, the power to choose, so when you gain the knowledge of the 'what' and the 'where' of vitamins, you also gain the power to use it. With this you can choose health and happiness—and your life is now your choice.

Each step is a thirty-day, one-step-at-a-time plan, so focus on this and do it for thirty days, and then move on to the next step.

STEP TEN

SIMPLE STRETCHING

A while back I had a problem with my lower back. I am sixty-eight and I work out regularly, including sit-ups, outside of my dancing, and I have relatively good posture, so I was having a hard time figuring this out. I saw a chiropractor and then an osteopath, and we figured out that I had a leg injury a couple of years back and had become dependent on the other leg to the extent that I became off balance. The osteopath showed me a couple of stretching exercises to do to get back to balance, and right away after the first exercise the pain started to go away.

I started to think, 'if this is good for my back, maybe it could be good for my whole body'; so I joined a Bikram yoga class for a short time. I then decided to (because of my travel) to put together my own workout stretching system based on my personal needs, so I did, and my back kept improving, and at this point the back pain is fast becoming history. What I noticed is that over a six-month or so period not only was my back getting better, but another problem also disappeared—I'd had stiff joints and shoulder pain, and it was a job just bending down to tie my shoe, but this all just disappeared.

So now I am understanding it all. As I look around me I find a lot of people who are in that same boat, but it is not so hard to understand. It's simple: use it or lose it. When you don't use your muscles they become small and weak and don't support your skeletal system, which in turn puts stress on your joints because the muscle is not supporting them, so you wind up with joint pain and stiffness, and also back and other problems. You then become very susceptible to falling and other real problems like broken bones.

When you start to stretch your muscles and make them stronger, you start to move better and lose those aches and pains that a lot of people consider a normal consequence of aging, but the truth is that it probably has a lot more to do with what you are eating and drinking than anything else. So step number ten is to incorporate 15–30 minutes of stretching into each day, and you will find that all of the stiffness, aches, and joint pain will disappear.

IN THE PLACE WHERE YOU FIND

YOURSELF YOU FIND EVERYONE ELSE

IN YOUR LIFE

IF I COULD, I CAN

Who are you, what do you think, how do you feel, what do you do, how do you do it, what do you like, what do you dislike, how do you live, where do you live, how do you see yourself, how do other people see you, what's most important in your life, what would you change, what would you do differently if you could?

Take about ten minutes, read the questions one at a time standing in front of a mirror, and answer as if your entire life depended on that answer. Then from those heartfelt answers act as if your life depended on it and do what you decided. You are probably saying that if it were so easy to do I would do it and would have already— the truth is I could be an atheist today and a total believer in God tomorrow, or I could be a butcher today and a nomadic biker tomorrow, I could be a teacher today and a Buddhist monk tomorrow, I could be a librarian today and an exotic dancer tomorrow, a prostitute today and a nun tomorrow, a dog trainer today and a race car driver tomorrow, a housewife today or a great comedian tomorrow, a street beggar or president.

The first thought to follow is that it is not possible to change that way and so quickly, but before you finish that thought ask yourself this: If you are a smoker who "can't quit" and you were put in a gas-filled room every time you had the urge to light up, and you knew that it would turn you and everything in the room into ashes, would you smoke? If you have an "unconscious habit" that you want to change but can't, ask yourself if every time I did this someone would take off one of my fingers, would you still be doing it?

The point is that you haven't given yourself the right reason or the need to change (your habits are still wandering free). Change truly is only a thought away. If you truly decided and totally focused on it right, the change would happen now. The saying goes that "you always hurt the one you love, the one you shouldn't hurt at all" or "familiarity breeds contempt." It may be true that the ones we love, who are closest to us, are often the target of our dissatisfaction, whereas strangers and friends are often only allowed to see the best of us ... why? Because you keep making that decision, and as a result are not giving yourself the will or need to change, once you *truly* decide that the rest of your life will be different (a true and conscious decision) and give yourself a reason that leaves you no other choice, then it happens. For example, we don't want our friends or other people to think that we are strange, unhappy, or not so nice, so we *act* differently, and at that point in time we keep making the choice to act differently, because we want them to see us as nice, happy, and friendly. But if we give ourselves the need, we could act that way with everyone (the mind doesn't know the difference between acting and being), and the habit would ingrain itself.

Jesus said, "These things I do you can do them and more," so you do have the power to wake up to anything you choose to do, be, or become. So take a serious moment to give yourself the right reasons, and wake up tomorrow as the beautiful person you want to be, enjoying the life you choose.

You can.

ALL THAT YOU COULD EVER WANT

HAS ALREADY BEEN CREATED

FOR YOU.

YOU ONLY NEED

TO FAITHFULLY

OPEN YOUR HANDS

AND REACH OUT.

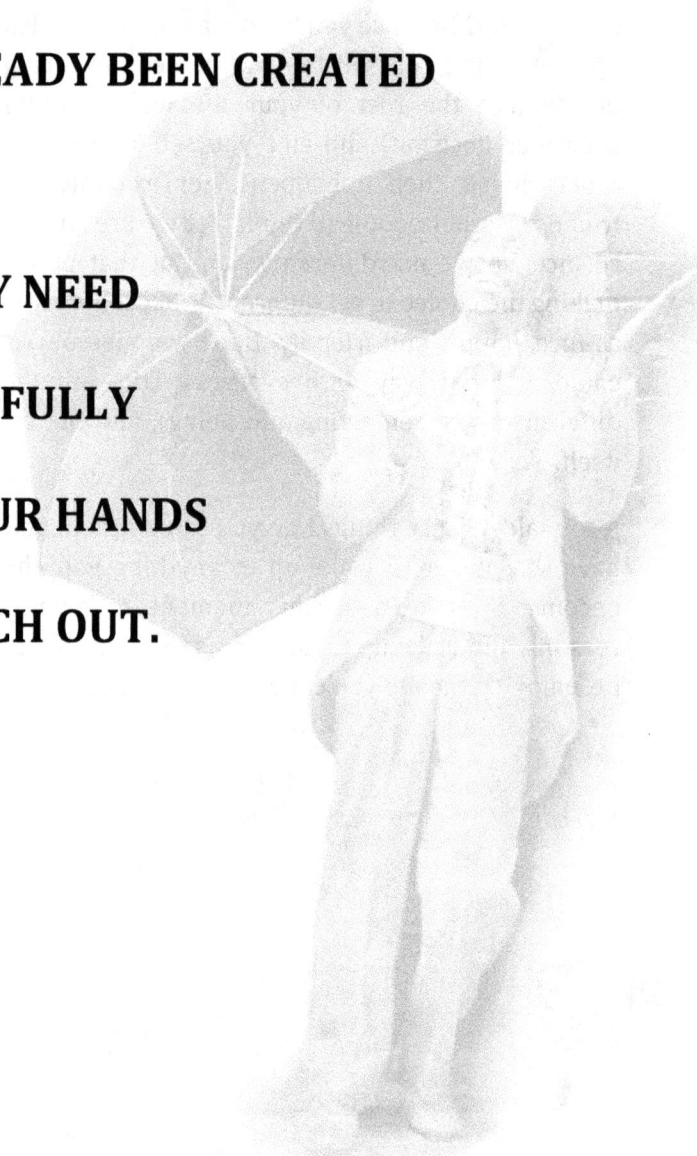

SIMPLE EXERCISE

Exercise without exercising—this may sound crazy, but it makes a lot of sense if you just think about it a little. Anything that you do that requires movement can be slightly modified to benefit you as exercise. It can begin with getting up in the morning and putting your underwear on.

Try this: first grab each side of your underwear as if you are going to step into them, then go to the bed and fall back (with your underwear still held in both hands) on the bed bringing both feet up at the same time, then stick both feet through the opening in the underwear at the same time, then when you roll back forward you can stand up with your underwear on. Next, put your socks on this way one leg at a time, then put your pants on the same way with both legs at the same time.

Now you are dressed and ready for the shoes. Bend your knees to pick up one shoe, then stand up and pick up the same leg high enough to put your foot in the shoe. Then put one foot in front of the other and bend your knees to tie your shoe, and then put the other shoe on the same way. It may take you a few times to get used to the bending and stretching, but the more you do it the easier it gets, and the more flexible and conditioned you get.

If you walk to get the bus, try leaving at the same time but fast walking to the next stop beyond the one you usually go to.

If you drive to work, park your car further away from your destination, then walk fast to get there (if you are female and it is dark it is safer to park as close to the door as possible). Do the same thing when you go shopping or to do other things. Also get in the habit of taking the stairs. If there are a lot of stairs, do this whenever you have to go in or out; if there as just a few stairs, try going up and down them two or three times if possible.

Lastly, if you find yourself standing in line from time to time, just do the first step from the TIH workout (step number one, the walk step). In a short time you will see a lot of your aches, pains, stiffness, and stress go away.

WHATEVER I HAVE CAN BENEFIT ME, BUT ONLY IF I MAKE THE CHOICE TO USE IT.

SIMPLE FACTS

"Kill the head and the body will follow." This is the simple strategy that Muhammad Ali (who is considered the greatest boxer of all time) employed, and it is the same tactic that many parents have used (unknowingly and due to their own insecurity) on their children, to greatly hinder or sometimes destroy the life of the child.

From the time that he knew that he would box another person, Muhammad Ali would begin his psychological barrage, telling his opponent how incapable he was, or how stupid he was, or how ugly he was, that he was not smart enough, and so on. For news and promotion reasons the two boxers were constantly meeting in public, so they could keep hearing these things before the match. Ali's purpose was that if you tell another person a particular thing enough (even if their common sense tells them it's not true), they will start to react to this.

By the time they actually got in the ring with him they were so angry (because their insecurity told them that some or all of this was true) that they would defeat themselves—he only had to finish the job physically. Why? Because they had basically lost their mind (their ability to think rationally due to anger). In other words, kill the brain and the body will follow.

Now think about your health and happiness. If they are not at the center of your thinking and reasoning they have been compromised, and are in need of correction.

To do this you must first understand that faith and habit are the masters of change, if you believe in anything enough it becomes your reality, as thought is the parent of reality in this life.

If you do anything enough it becomes habit (your basic truth and reality), and can go on working seemingly without thought.

You can believe that God created everything and that and that anything that you want or need (life, health, and happiness) is available here for you. Then you only need to live your purpose and share it with the world to be healthy and happy.

Another word on habit: If you do anything enough your brain accepts it as a part of your reality, and allows it to continue regardless of whether it hurts or helps your cause for life.

This is to say that we need to stop killing our brain and start to feed it positive thoughts until this practice becomes habit for you and your life.

Your habits should be only those things that serve your health and happiness, and what you want will become yours.

Now, today is your opportunity to think, reason, and go forward into a life of health and happiness.

THE ONLY THING PERMANENT IS

CHANGE AND NOTHING

IN THE UNIVERSE CAN AVOID THIS,

YOUR CHOICE IN THIS IS HOW YOU

WILL CHANGE

SIMPLE DIETS

How many times have you heard the statement "Diets don't work"? Probably more than you would care to think about at this time. Well it's true, diets don't work.

Why? Because you are trying to fix a long-term problem with a short-term solution.

One of the main reasons that diets don't work is because people don't work at them. Why? Because although you may convince yourself that it's something that you can do for a short time, you already know that you will not keep doing it, because quitting at a certain point is already in the plan from the start.

If change and you start to do something (or eat something) for a short time, say two months, or up to a year, and then you stop and resume doing what you were doing before you made the change, then you are likely to go back to what you were before you made the change, because from the beginning you already understand that this change (diet) is not something you plan to continue. That in itself is the problem-temporary change can only get temporary results.

So it is better you forget about diets and focus on health and happiness with things that you can spend the rest of your life doing—a lifestyle change.

We are creatures of habit. And our first thought should be to become conscious of our desires. No matter what it is, you must be able to put your finger on what you want.

Then you can focus your attention on it (consciously) until it becomes habit and you don't have to make a big effort to focus on it.

The real commitment is a lifelong commitment to lifestyle change (not just a temporary fix on an old lifestyle), simply because what your lifestyle has been up to now has not worked to get you what and where you want to be in your life up to this point.

This is where TIH comes in. TIH is a lifestyle plan for life; it is something that you could easily see yourself doing the rest of your life, without a problem.

TIH is a plan you can live with in health and happiness.

JUST REMEMBER, WE LIVE THE DAYS
OF OUR LIVES ONE AT A TIME, SO
THAT IS HOW WE CHANGE IT... ONE
DAY, ONE THING AT A TIME.

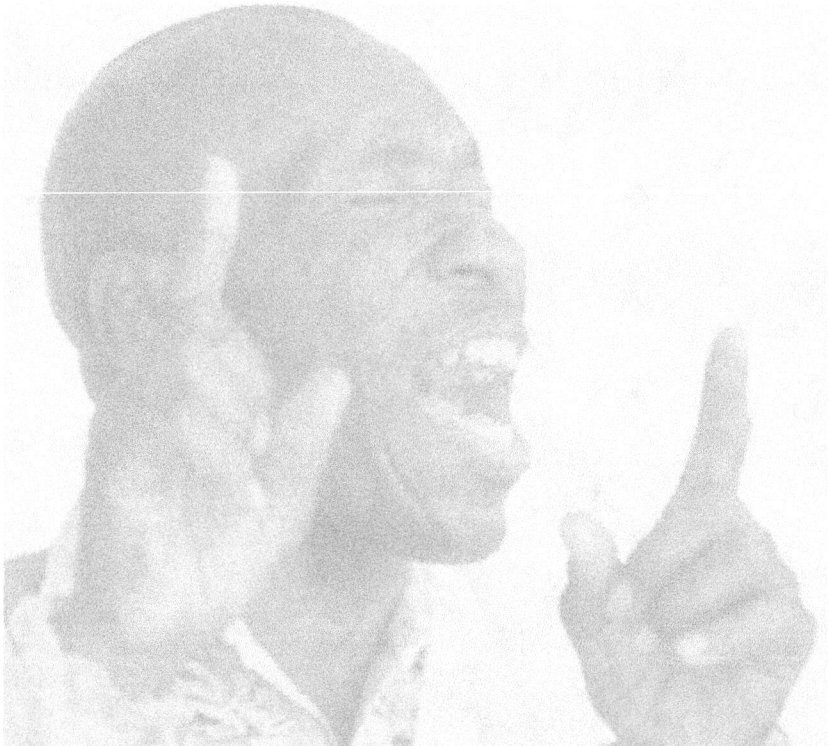

SIMPLE EATING

"It is not so much what you are eating, as what's eating you." God and the universe create in nature abundance and perfection, so all that you need in the way of fresh fruits and vegetables, if left to grow uninhibited by man, will rejuvenate again and again to be available for us to eat.

Our problem arises because we fail to seek what we consume in our lives from the source (such as fresh fruits and vegetables), because this is the place where they serve us totally and completely.

Man with his limited understanding has not the ability to compete with or to improve upon nature, and it is the nature of the human body to constantly heal itself, seeking to return to wholeness. When we do anything to hinder that work, the body begins to speak to us in the way of sickness, pain, and disease, And if we continue what we're doing and continue to ignore it, the body starts to shut down one part to keep another part going; and if still ignored, it will cease to do its work completely because you have deprived it of its means—so it stops and you stop.

Often during this process we began to seek out doctors and suchlike to heal us, but as Jesus said, "You are healed by your faith." The doctor may only be a factor in postponing your demise, because you need to come around to the fact that your body was made to function properly on what the earth provides the way it provides it. Sickness and disease may be more of what you are doing to yourself than what is being done to you, and only you have the power to change that. Just as the mind plays a big part in sickness, it also plays a big part in healing. If you believe that nature provides us, then your mind will lead you to think about and to eat what is right for you.

It is ironic that when you are sick and you go to the hospital that they give you salad, fruit, and vegetables mostly, when if they gave you the information that you should eat this, you maybe would not have to go to the hospital to begin with.

I have seen firsthand relatives and friends, who upon being told that they had a terminal illness, switched to fresh fruit and vegetables and juice and plain old water, and then returned to the doctor from four months to a year later to find no sign of the illness.

So you can start a life of health and happiness by taking time to examine what you are eating while you are eating it, and determine if it is really serving your nutritional needs. If not, start to eliminate piece by piece and replace it with something that does.

Just remember, we live the days of our lives one day at a time, so that is how we change it—one thing at a time.

You are here and alive, so you still have the time.

WHEN YOU STOP USING YOUR BODY,

YOU START LOSING YOUR BODY.

SIMPLE RULE

FOR HEALTH AND HAPPINESS

Healthy people are happy people and happy people are healthy people—it all begins with finding yourself.

You begin by asking, "What do I like about myself, and what would I like to change about myself to what I like?" This is a question about you and your life; it is also a question about what's in your life.

Take a look at everything in and of your life, starting today, one day at a time, one situation at a time.

This puts you on the right road, because in the end these questions are about your life, and start you up the ladder to health and happiness.

You must remember that where you are physically and mentally is where you have chosen to be through a series of choices and decisions. Say if you are overweight, it is you that is making the choice to be that way by either overeating or eating improperly, or not getting enough exercise, or all of the above. The decision to be or do anything is a decision that must be made day by day.

We get up and we keep trying to repeat what we did yesterday, but the realization is that we can't. The whole universe and everything in it is constantly changing - the only thing permanent is change. Your only choice is how you will change. This is your choice, and every day you wake up you have that choice available to you. You must take full responsibility for what you have because you have created it through thought and action.

So there is no need to blame anyone or anything for the circumstances of your life, what you like or dislike. It's all yours. Look at it, take responsibility for it, and then you can change it.

No matter who you are, where you are, or what you do, the one chance you have for change is yourself, by first accepting what you have, then deciding what you want, then giving your attention to that day by day.

Remembering that health and happiness are a thought first (the origin of life): the decision, then implementation.

To truly change you must only give your time and attention to that which you want (ignore the rest and it will go away). This is the place where you find health and happiness.

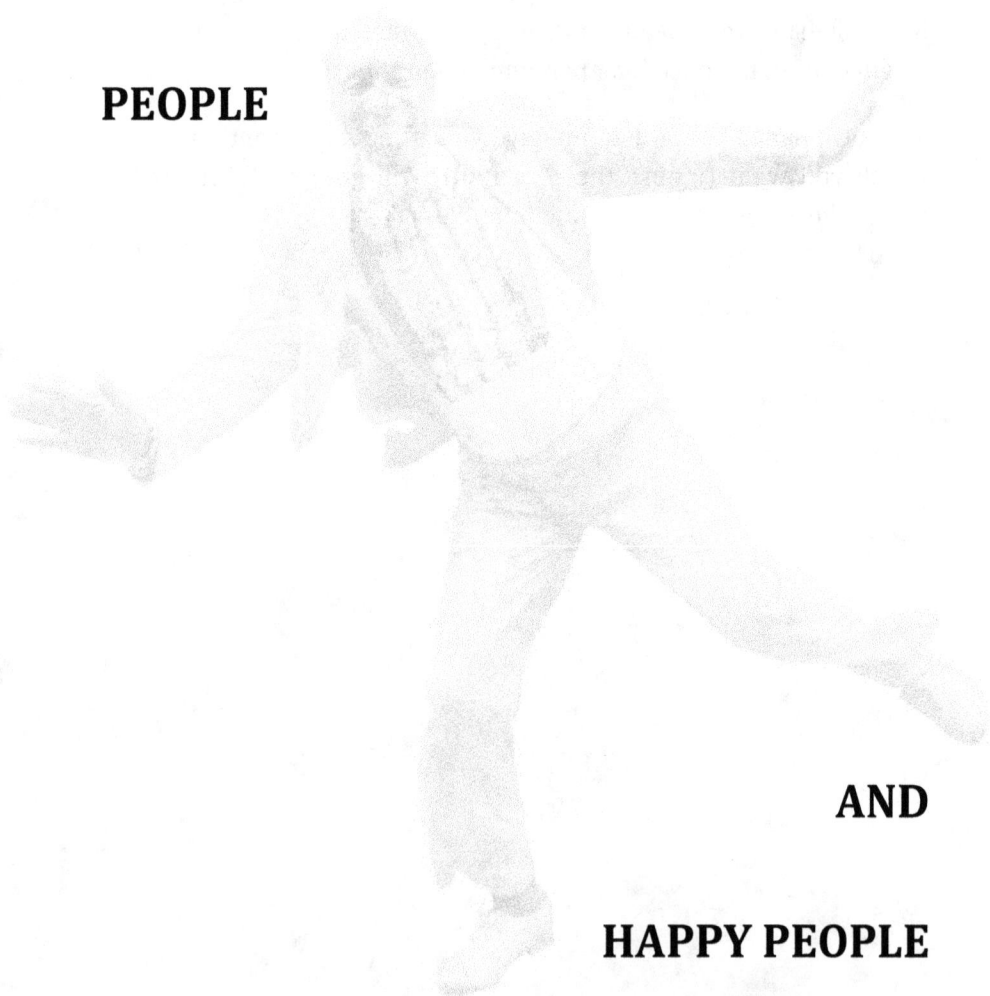

HEALTHY PEOPLE

ARE HAPPY

PEOPLE

AND

HAPPY PEOPLE

ARE HEALTHY PEOPLE

SIMPLE BODY

Your body is designed for your life, and just like everything else in life it should be used for its designed purpose.

All movable parts should be moved every day—arms, legs, neck, and so on—they need movement to sustain their capacity to move.

The old saying "If you don't use it, you lose it" is very true of your mind, your body, and your life. I recommend at least one half hour of aerobic (TIH) workout and the same if not more of stretching or flexibility training. The benefits can often be seen through your energy level, feeling of well-being, and a simple comparison with the people around you who are your age. But don't do any of this, and you see the difference.

You could consider this as "me time," and for your life and well-being everyone should have me time everyday if possible.

Doing this works for your whole system: your brain (oxygen helps you think better), circulation (your blood flows better), your immune system (when germs attack, your immune system mounts a defense against them; usually your temperature goes up), your heart (with increased blood flow your heart gets more oxygen and performs better), and so on—everything works better when it is used for its designed purpose.

So you look better, feel better, think better, and most important you get in touch with your body with an important message: that you care about your body (and your life).This helps you live beyond sickness and disease.

Make this practice a habit and your body will be like a good soldier, always at its highest fighting level against disease, sickness, and accidents.

BUILD THE BODY THAT YOU WOULD

LIKE TO SEE AND LIVE IN

SIMPLE CHANGE

The simple truth is that we think ourselves into health and happiness, because if you don't first have the thought you cannot have the experience, which is the subject of the thought and your life.

There are two basic things required for change, decision and intention. No matter what it is that you have in your life, everything you do either adds to your life (love and happiness), or it takes away. The decision to eat adds to your life, the decision not to eat takes away from your life, so at some point in your life you made a conscious decision to eat. Everything else is your life is the same: what you eat, how you eat, when you eat, and so on; it first had to be a thought, and then the action followed.

Conscious thought followed by action is the rule for success.

The process of change begins with becoming aware of what you have or what you have created (everything that you have in your life up till this point is what you have created from thought).

So you must ask yourself, "Does what I am thinking, what I am saying, or what I am doing really serve my life in the best way?" If not, then it's time for you to sit down and write out a plan for health and happiness, or your avenue to change.

Acceptance (of what you have and what you have created) is the first part; this allows you to set the stage for change (movement towards what you really want).This is the place where you remove the obstacles that you have created so that you can clearly see the way.

The usual obstacles are people, places, situations, and things (a relationship, job, money, house, or location). The problem is that we think that when any or all of these things change then we will, but it will never happen while you are waiting in unhappiness; it will only happen when you change, because you are the nucleus of change in life. Your life or situation depends on you for change.

You should know that everything that you do affects everything else that you will do. Or, when you change one part of anything, everything else that's a part of that thing must change or adjust to deal with the change.

The idea that change must happen outside of you first is the illusion that stands in front of happiness.

Your life will only and always follow the route of your thought, so think and decide and live.

CONSCIOUS THOUGHT FOLLOWED

BY ACTION

IS THE RULE FOR SUCCESS

SIMPLE HEALTH

"An ounce of prevention is worth a pound of cure." "Your food should be your medicine and your medicine should be your food." "We should eat to live, not live to eat."

You have probably heard one or more of these before, and if you are reading this right now, you are at the point of wanting to understand what your health is all about.

There is a part in the Bible that essentially says that every man is responsible for his own salvation. This covers your health and happiness, which means what you eat, how you eat, how much you eat, and what you feel, say, and do about things, because all of these have a bearing on your health and happiness.

We have access to a very large variety of foods (when I speak of food I am talking about what Mother Nature produces). God and the universe have assured that anything that you could want or need for life is available.

This is to simply say that fresh fruits and vegetables are your best source for life, so you should get them, preferably from the source (this means to gather them from the place where they grow).

Most sickness and disease can be traced back to simple nutritional deficiency. I believe this because I have experienced healing through simple nutrition.

So your best bet for a life of health and happiness should be planned around what you eat, drink, and think, because any problem you could have will be found in one or all three of these areas.

Your eating should involve understanding what and why you are eating.

Learn and eat, then eat and learn, until it becomes habit. The habit of health and happiness.

WHAT YOU EAT, DRINK AND THINK IS

THE SIMPLEST ROAD TO HEALTH AND

HAPPINESS

SIMPLE HEARING

Sickness is simply body language—your body is telling you that you have not given it enough of what it needs to maintain health, or that you have depleted too much of what you had to maintain health.

This is the language of the body; every headache, every pain, every backache, leg, or foot ache, every upset stomach, everything that happens is like a red flag saying, "Come to see what is happening here."

Your body was created to function perfectly for all purposes.

Your mind is the computer, or the place where your body gets its functioning blueprint. It is always turned on but it should also be tuned in or conscious, which suggests that staying healthy means staying conscious.

Getting healthy and happy and staying that way is just another way of saying, "Stay present and conscious." If you are not, then you know from where your problems with health and happiness arise.

In the world we live in and the world we grow in, consciousness is not a common thing, even though at birth it is totally present, so we have to reprogram ourselves to get back to this. A good way to start is with 'me' time, this is a time when you are consciously living in the moment and aware of your body and how it is speaking to you; this can be a time you take every day to relax and to listen to yourself and your life.

Why is this so important? Because it is a vital link to health and happiness. Simply having the body and mind connection can determine how long you live, how well you stay, the quality of your life, how well you function physically, and everything that you do with yourself and others.

Everything that you get in life will cost you something in time, effort, or money. The time you spend to get in touch with your body will cost you such a small amount compared to the payoff.

An easy way to think of it is learning to walk a new way; at first it may seem a little awkward until you start to allow the habit to set in. Then you get fit for life, because in the end health and happiness are two of the most important things to have in life.

"YOUR BODY IS GOD'S TEMPLE", THE

TEMPLE IS A SOURCE OF KNOWLEDGE,

LISTEN TO YOUR BODY.

SIMPLE FIX

Where you are physically and mentally is a result of everything that you have done in your life up until this point. It doesn't matter if it is your weight, health, money, or happiness, this is as true for you as it is for everyone else.

Every thought that you have, every word that you speak, and every action that you do moves you towards where you are and how you are today, here and now .

If you are unhappy about yourself or anything in your life, you have no chance to change it until you first take full responsibility for creating it. Then you have the power, the power to change it. Otherwise, if you keep doing what you are doing (which got you to where you are today), you will keep getting what you are getting.

The very first rule of physical or mental change begins with your thinking. Every thought that you have will at some point play its way out in your life—that's what creating good or bad is all about.

Your thinking (the Bible says, "As a man thinketh, so is he") is at the center of everything you say, feel, and do, all the way down to who you are.

Try this simple experiment to help you to understand this. First think of a situation that was very unhappy for you. When you are fully there in the thought and feeling of this memory, at that moment try to be happy at the same time; it simply doesn't work.

Now think of a situation that made you feel very happy. Mentally return to that situation to totally feel it, then at this moment try to be unhappy; it also doesn't work, because where the thought goes, so does the rest of you.

What you should understand is that you have the power to create your life every moment of every day through positive or negative thinking.

It doesn't matter who you are or what you are at this point, that can change with the next thought.

So, life is a simple fix—if you want to be happy, you have to think happy thoughts and look for the good in every situation, and if you want to be healthy, you start with healthy thoughts; if you want to be rich, you have to start with rich thoughts, and make these thoughts the center of your focus.

So read this, focus on and understand this, and you will have found the foundation for having what you want in life.

YOU HAVE THE POWER TO CREATE
YOUR LIFE EVERY MOMENT OF EVERY
DAY THROUGH POSITIVE OR
NEGATIVE THINKING.

SIMPLE LAUGHTER

Laughter is food for the soul, or, happy leads to healthy and healthy leads to happy. Laughter makes you feel better not just mentally but physically as well. It is one of the greatest antidepressants (it chases away unhappy thoughts). You may think, "How can I laugh? Look at me, look at my life, look at my situation, what could be funny about that?" Well that's the job of getting to happy; in fact, I laugh sometimes when I see myself and others taking life so seriously.

What can be confusing to some people is that they think that you cannot be serious if you laugh, but what it simply means is that you can be serious and feel good at the same time, and that's what you want.

During slavery black people established laughter as a means of survival, and if you hang out with Black people, no matter what their situation looks like, they can often find a reason to laugh. They make jokes about the simplest and the smallest things just to have a reason to laugh. I look through books like *Readers Digest* to find short jokes and amusement that are spread throughout the book; I am always listening for a good joke.

I have a blind friend who will twist your words into something funny. I think this takes the boringness out of not having the sense of vision for him. As for me, this is a part of my feeling good about life while I am getting on with living.

There are joke books you can buy, there are books with titles like "Laugh Your Way to Health," and so on, to show you how important laughter can be. There was a famous book author who, after being diagnosed with cancer, went into the hospital and ordered all of the funny movies that he could get and watched them over and over and laughed until he was cured.

Laughter is anti-stress, anti-disease, anti-anything that doesn't make you feel good in life. The point is life is serious, but it is also funny if you look and you just find what you look for in life. So an important part of your life should be laughter for health and happiness.

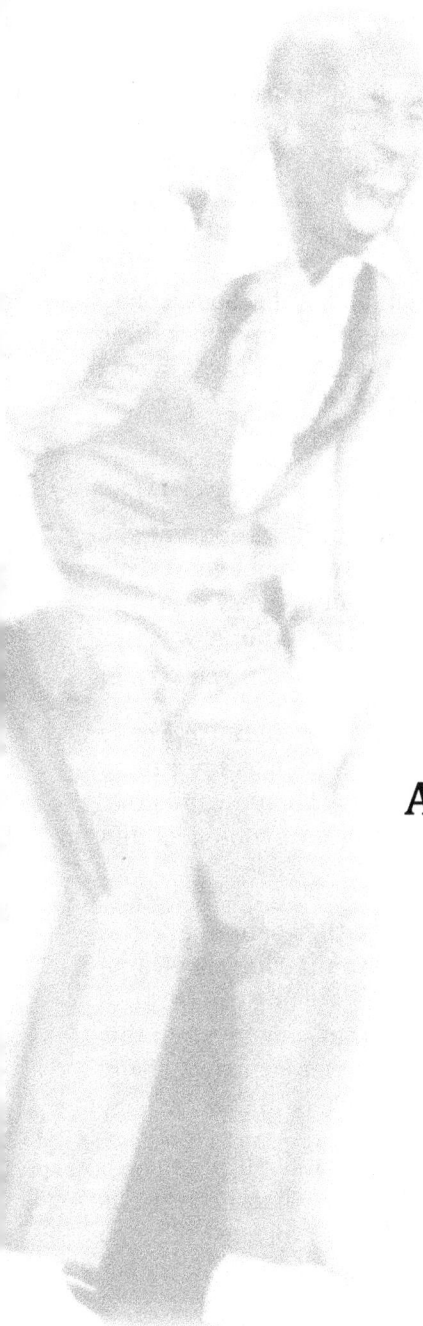

LAUGHTER

IS THE BEST FOOD

FOR THE SOUL,

WHEN YOU LAUGH

EVERYTHING

ABOUT YOU AND IN YOU

FEELS GOOD.

SIMPLE LIFE

I was shopping for a good printer, so I walked into a print shop once and was greeted by what I would now describe as a wonderful soul. This lady came shining out from the back of the shop, and from her first words, "How are you? What can I do for you today?" I felt that she had already made me a lifetime customer. I asked about printing and copying, and she began to take me through the possibilities for what I wanted (all of this was just preliminary, because I had already decided from her first words that I would get my work done there). I hung out maybe a little longer than necessary (it was such a pleasant experience), and then I went out of there feeling really great.

As I climbed into my car and sat for a moment, I began to think, "Why did I feel so good dealing with this person? It wasn't that she was exceptional looking or anything like that." And then I got it. This lady was doing what she loved to do. It came out in every way; she was living her purpose, doing what she was born to do; it was her calling.

I related so much to this lady and the way she was because I have the same way with what I do. I am an entertainer; it is my calling (and I heeded the call). I love to hear about it, talk about it, and do it. It's not work for me, it is joy, and I think that other people feel that from me for that reason.

One of the biggest downfalls of our times is that people are not encouraged enough to follow their calling or to do what they came here to do, so we have working just to make a living, or because they want to make money, or they were told that they must do this or that to be accepted in this life. All of this can steer you away from yourself and your purpose and reason for being here in this life.

Sometimes we have many excuses for not living our purpose, such as, when this or that happens then I can start, or when I reach this place I can start—no matter what the reason they all say the same thing: tomorrow. But we all know by now that tomorrow never comes, or as the Bible says, "We are not promised tomorrow."

Not living your cause or purpose is one of the root causes of unhappiness in our society, including unhappiness, depression, relationship problems, disease, hostility, anger, money problems, and it can be linked directly to most anything that does not work well in your life.

This is why I suggest taking inventory of your all-around happiness level. If it is in the negatives, then this should be one of the first places you look at and start doing something about now. Even if you only have the thought right now, that is the beginning of the plan to freedom. Remember, diligence is the price of freedom.

You must persist in getting the life you want, where your job, purpose, and reason for life can be seen in one place: You.

When you get to this point (of living your purpose), not only do you reach happiness in yourself, but everyone around you will share in that happiness, and the whole world becomes a better place because of you.

"IF YOU LOVE WHAT YOU DO FOR A LIVING, YOU MAY NEVER WORK A DAY IN YOUR LIFE"

SIMPLE ASKING

THE MORE YOU ASK THE MORE YOU GET

Often in our lives we act as victims of circumstances, when the real truth is we are the victims of our own created circumstances. There is one simple way to began eliminating this from your life: just ask for what you want.

If you want a certain car, to feel a certain way, to do a certain thing, to have a great relationship with whomever, to eat a certain food, to live in a certain place, to have nice flowers, to look a certain way, to meet certain people, to be happy and healthy, and so on, just ask. That's the first and most important step.

When you ask you affirm your faith in God, in the universe, in life, in others, and in yourself, that you can have what you want, because at that point you actually put the fear of not having behind you, and you put the whole universe on notice, because the action has started.

An easy way to understand this is to understand that anything and everything in the entire universe has an effect on everything else; one breath from you causes the air around you to change, so the air all over also has to change, however slightly.

One of the most powerful tools for completion in your life is simple asking. If you would begin every step with the phrase "This is what I would like", then you are already at the point where you have nothing to lose (because you don't have it), and everything to gain (what you are asking for).

This covers any and all situations and things in and around your life. Never take for granted that anyone knows what you want or would like to happen, because quite often no matter who they are, they don't. When you ask, you and everyone else know exactly what you want, and that's a good thing.

The fear of asking stands in front of the fear of having. You only need to know that f-e-a-r is only "false evidence appearing real";

knowing this allows you to put fear behind you and faith in front of you.

And by faith, the more you ask the more you will receive, and the more you receive, the more you can ask.

So from the most menial to the most elaborate and all in between, your success in getting depends on your willingness to ask.

Most people at some point began to recognize those things that they feel would make their lives better for them; unfortunately ninety-nine percent of them just didn't ask, for whatever reason—because there is no good reason or excuse, only fear tells you there is.

You deserve the best that this life has to offer you; we all do. We only need to take responsibility for this. The Bible says, "Ask and it shall be given," "Seek and you shall find"—it's all another way to say, "Ask for what you want."

So get the habit of asking, keep the habit of asking, and learn to live comfortably with it; it is your human right, which begins with asking.

The final note is this: sometimes you ask, and life asks you in return if you are sincere. Sometimes the way it does this is by having you ask again and sometimes again; sincere people understand that "No" only means that you need to ask again—someone else, somewhere else, or in another way—because every time you ask the wrong person, you are getting closer to the right person.

Success is apparent to those who ask in sincerity.

"ASK AND IT SHALL BE GIVEN", "SEEK AND YEE SHALL FIND"

SIMPLE FOCUS

You buy a very expensive camera and you begin to take pictures—picture after picture, after picture, after picture. At some point you begin to notice, *I have lots of (otherwise) nice pictures, but ninety percent are not clear*; the subject is too far, too close or blurry. So you go to the person who develops the pictures and you say, "Hey, I got this expensive camera and I am taking all of these nice pictures, but they are not coming out right. What are you doing to my pictures?" That person says to you, "I am only developing what you give me. That's all I can do." After a couple of rounds the person developing your pictures asks you to bring in your camera. He takes a look at it and he agrees that it is an expensive and good camera, so he asks you to tell him what you do. "I just point and shoot," you explain. He then explains, "OK, you have the right camera and you are doing the right thing, but you need the right lens that will focus automatically on the subject." You reply, "Oh, so that's my problem." So you go out and you buy the right lens for your camera, and as before you just point and shoot, but unlike before, with the right lens you find that ninety-five to a hundred percent of your pictures are coming out good. Why? Because you are now focusing on the subject.

Can it be the same with your life? How focused are you on what you want and what you want your life to be? Happiness, love, success, peace of mind, money—or do you even know what it is that you want? If the answer is no, then you make the decision (buy a camera and the right lens), and then allow that decision to become conscious habit in your mind (a habit is simply a point of focus repeated over and over until it becomes automatic).

We have a lot of these things in our (mind) life that we really don't want or need, things that simply get in the way of our focusing on what we really want. As a result, being unfocused becomes the habit. Things like resentment towards those who have what we want, excuses like, "I don't know" or "I don't know how," fear of true success (a big one) or preoccupation with (otherwise irrelevant) other things, or the sad belief that we can't have what we want (must be changed to "I can have what I want").

These are examples of our picture being out of focus. So we must first, stop blaming the developer (other people, places, things, and situations) for our problem; next, go back into our mind (the store or storehouse) and decide what we really want (the proper lens); and then point and shoot, point and shoot, and our hopes, dreams, and desires will become our life (clear pictures).

It is *" he who believes that it is so that opens the gate, topples the mountain or calms the sea, for there is no stronger element in your life than your belief "*.

YOUR WHOLE LIFE IS A CONSCIOUS

DECISION, YOU ONLY NEED TO

BECOME CONSCIOUS OF IT.

SIMPLE LOVE

"Love thy neighbor as thyself" means that you have to first have the love in order to be able to share it. It means that you have a healthy portion of self-love not selfless love to give to another, or what I would like to call finding God in yourself and your situations.

The problem can arise when you don't have for yourself what you are attempting to give away to others.

A lack of self-love can be a source of many (if not all) problems in your life, things like war, killing, fighting, deceit, unhappiness, sickness, anger, marriage problems, disease, bad career, unhappy relationship, and so on—everything you do is affected by the way you feel about yourself.

Love is actually not something that we can give away; it is only something that we can share, and to share it you have to have it.

Love is of vital importance in this life—I mean self-love—and a lack of it is one of the vital causes of breakdown in our society. I would say that most if not all of the problems that you could have in this life could be eliminated through self-love.

When you love yourself, it is not like you hold false pride in yourself that has nothing to do with love. What has to do with love is when you can look and see how you feel, which is good, because you intentionally think, feel, say, and do things that help you to feel good. You have a positive attitude about yourself, you do and work at things that feel good to you, your self-esteem is high, you like yourself, and physically as well as mentally you take care of yourself totally. The good thing is that you not only have all of this, but you have all of this to share (love radiates), because your knowing how it feels to be loved, allows you to identify how it feels coming from and going to others. When you love yourself there is always a place inside of you that feels warm; this is the essence of self-love for you and every one you come into contact with in your life.

So if you feel that there is something missing from your life, start to look in the place of self-love first, and answer that call for self-love inside of you. Then you will see the beauty that life can take on around you.

ONCE YOU FIND A REASON FOR LIFE,

YOU CAN BEGIN TO LIVE WITH THE

REASON THAT YOU'VE FOUND.

SIMPLE MAGIC

(The Magic of Music for Health and Happiness)

I was recently watching a documentary about a nursing home that was experimenting with music therapy. One particular elderly gentleman was suffering from Alzheimer's disease. He was slumped over in a wheelchair and seemed to be unaware of who and where he was, so they began to play some big band music with energy in it. You could see him straighten up in his wheelchair, open his eyes, and start to talk coherently about the music and the people who made it, and he eventually started to sing along in tune with the music.

I thought, "This is the real power of music, the power to transform, because it touches a special part of you".

I have been in entertainment most of my life, and this is one of the first things that a true entertainer learns. When I feel good I look good, when I look good I think and act good; a complete circle.

If you don't believe me, put on an energetic song that you really like and see how energetic you start to feel.

First any negative or unhappy thoughts seem to go away, as your whole body starts to feel energetic.

Music actually changes the molecular structure of the air around you and puts energy into the air.

Your whole system works. Even if you are sitting down and listening to music, you start to burn energy, and in the process you lose fat and build muscle. The more you intentionally subject yourself to energetic music, by listening, singing, dancing, or working out, the higher your energy level goes, so your energy from what you are doing can increase or double.

That is the main point of TIH—it's not likely that you will ever see a fat tap dancer.

LOVE IS ACTUALLY NOT SOMETHING
THAT WE CAN GIVE AWAY; IT IS ONLY
SOMETHING THAT WE CAN SHARE,
AND TO SHARE IT YOU HAVE TO FIRST
HAVE IT.

SIMPLE WAYS

To be 20-30 percent Healthier and Happier almost Overnight

It is of the utmost importance to know how to be happy and healthy, and it is as important to know what not to do to be healthy and happy.

The simple rule is that it's either good for you or it's not. If it adds to you happiness, health, and well-being, then it's good for you (food for thought), and if it doesn't add to your happiness, health, and well-being, then it's not good for you (also food for thought), and it needs to be avoided and never looked back on again.

My rule for this is anytime I find something that I am doing that does not work for my health and happiness, I immediately start to look for something that does to replace it. We are creatures of habit, and to simply stop doing or thinking something that does not work for us leaves a space or a hole in our lives; so if we don't put something there to fill that hole, the old habit will return to fill it. Drugs, alcohol, smoking, unhappiness are all addictive, which means that they have become habit and now the habit is in control of your doing, not you.

Anything in your life can be changed. The first thing to do is to acknowledge it; that is the beginning of change. Then say to yourself (aloud), "I am responsible for anything that happens in, of, and to my life. No other person, place, situation, or thing, only me." By the act of accepting this, you immediately feel and gain power over your life.

Now you are ready to go to work on your thinking and doing, always reminding yourself that if it feels good to think it, then it's good to do and is a part of my health and happiness, so I will look for more of these thoughts to reflect in my thinking, eating, and drinking. That replenishes my body and keeps me alive and healthy.

Than start a list of things to remove from your life one by one. Find replacements and move them into place—and don't look back. Find the bad habits and replace them.

LOSE YOURSELF IN MUSIC,

AND YOU WILL FIND YOURSELF IN

A GOOD PLACE

SIMPLE PLAN

"No plan is a plan to fail." You are the main subject of life—your dreams, your hopes, your desires spring from all that God could have in store for you.

Life—to be happy, to be healthy, to be rewarding, or to just be—requires a plan. This does not mean that you can predict the future by planning. If you have ever noticed, no matter how well you plan, what you want comes, but because of the many universal solutions that we are not aware of your plan comes in its own way. The plan is more for you to know where to focus your attention and energy.

Your life requires a plan. You make plans every day from moment to moment, but because it is happening unconsciously it's just a habit, so it feels like it's not happening because it's not an intentional, conscious plan.

Have you ever had someone say to you that you have to think about what you are doing? What they really mean is that you need to become conscious of what you are thinking and doing (a plan) in the moment.

If you have a broken leg, you have to make a new plan for tying your shoe, because the old plan does not work for the new situation. But when your leg is completely healed you have to plan on tying your shoe like you did before the broken leg, which could seem hard or awkward, but unless you become conscious of the moment and make a new plan now, you (as so often is the case for life) will keep doing things that do not really serve your will at that moment; in fact, you stay a step behind your life.

Happiness is a plan. More happiness is a better plan—to live in the moment of enjoyment of your life.

Yesterday is past, tomorrow only a possibility, today is what you have to plan now. With a conscious plan you essentially decide what the rest of your life will be about, so if it doesn't look good or feel good, just stay conscious.

Plan in the moment and re-plan. First give yourself a purpose (what you want), and then decide on the route to take to get to what you want—you now have a plan. Without a plan you leave your life to chance, not choice. Your plan is your choice.

"IT IS BETTER TO CHOOSE YOUR

HABITS THAN

ALLOWING YOUR HABITS

TO CHOOSE YOU"

SIMPLE PSYCHOLOGY

(Of happiness, health, and weight loss)

One hundred percent of who you are, how you are, what you are, how you look, how happy you are, and whatever happens to you from this point on comes from what you think and what you believe.

What I choose to think and believe has no choice but to become my reality. The most famous healer of all (Jesus) said to the people, "You are healed by your faith" (your faith is what you have chosen to believe). These were the words of Jesus, who took no credit for healing the people; he gave all the credit to them and their belief or faith.

Stop and look around you at everything you see, for without a thought, whatever you see could not exist.

At the beginning of every problem stands your belief in lies, deception, anger, unhappiness, and so on. Negative beliefs will ripple through your life, affecting everything you say, feel, and do— this is the very power of unhappy thinking or belief.

Someone said to me once that you can't always be happy. I asked, "Why? Where is it written or who decided that?" I am sometimes not as happy as I am at other times, but I am always happy. And the greatest aspect of this is what I call finding God (the good) in every situation.

Yes, God is always there. Believe this and look, and you will find him. As this becomes habit, you become happier, and a happy person is a healthy person. Why? Because your happiness feels so good that you are willing to do the work to stay there (taking care of your mind, body, and soul and that of others).

And that's life.

So look in the mirror and ask yourself, "Am I happy?" Honestly answer, and then sit down (make time; this is your life) and make a list of all the things in your life you have to be happy about. Then begin to put all of your attention on these things, and always be thankful for these things and the opportunity to have them in your life.

As you focus your attention on these things, you will find more things waiting to be acknowledged; as you acknowledge them there will come a time when that's all there is to acknowledge—you have the habit of happiness, and we all know that habits are not so easy to break.

So get the habit of happiness.

A SIMPLE CONSCIOUS PLAN NOW WILL

TELL YOU EVERYTHING

YOU NEED TO KNOW ABOUT

YOUR PAST PRESENT AND FUTURE

SIMPLE WORDS

When you think good, you feel good; when you feel good, you act good; when you act good, you look good; and when you look good, you feel good—life is presenting to you the perfect circle always.

Your life began from a good thought, and for you to proceed you must continue in the process.

"Ask and it shall be given," "Seek and you shall find."

As physical health is a big part of mental health, so mental health is a very big part of physical health.

Positive thinking attracts positive situations and positive results; negative thinking brings negative situations and negative results.

Another way to say this is to find good in every situation and let that becomes the focus of your attention and thought, so regardless of the situation you have to come out on the good end. Or, if you focus your attention on that which is bad or does not work for your life, then that is what you will see and get. Again, there is no way around the fact that we see what we look for.

"You are where your attention takes you."

One of the main keys to success in this life is simply to be nice, ask for what you want, don't yell, don't fight, don't argue, don't be afraid, don't be shy, just ask. Ask God, ask yourself, friends, your lover, your boss, anyone and everyone who will hear you, but ask. If you don't ask, no one knows, including you, so no one can respond.

So ask and give the universe something to work with on your behalf.

LIKE EVERYTHING ELSE IN YOUR LIFE

HAPPINESS IS A DECISION THAT YOU

MUST MAKE AND KEEP.

SIMPLE ACCOMPLISHMENT

Think it, feel it, say it (or ask it), do it. From the second you have the thought the universe around you begins to move to accommodate you and your thought, and from that point on, you and only you can stop it from becoming reality. If you have a thought and you don't follow through with the feeling associated with that thought, then you have begun to short-circuit your intentions. If you allow the feeling to complete its course unimpeded, the universe becomes even more receptive to the thought; at this point, to say it opens up the vibrational level of life for doing, and with each step the space for activation gets bigger until manifestation occurs. Your happiness and its level can only come from this place.

This is a simple test to tell you where your level of happiness is. Either stop whatever you are doing right now, or set aside a time to do this.

Take a look around you, and then pick out an object to focus on. No matter what it is, give it your full attention. Now find the beauty of its existence—it doesn't matter what it is—and then look for its designed purpose, its reason for creation, and whatever it is that makes it unique from any and everything else.

By now you are just looking at the beauty of nature and the glory of its work. How good do you now feel about this object? You have just given yourself good reason to feel good about this object and to feel good yourself. Now you feel good because you just found something good to feel good about. If this is not a part of what you do every day, in every situation, you understand now how to make happiness a habit, to have as much of it as you want.

Happiness is like anything else in your life, it is a choice and you have to choose it to have it. If you choose it enough then it becomes habit and continues on its own, and you have effectively become the author of your own happiness. It's simple, and if you want to do it the opportunity is always with you and your choosing.

AS PHYSICAL HEALTH IS A BIG PART

OF MENTAL HEALTH,

SO MENTAL HEALTH IS ALSO

A BIG PART OF PHYSICAL HEALTH.

SIMPLE TREATMENT

Changing ourselves and our lives can be as easy or as hard as we choose to make it. If you feel alone living in this world, you only have to know that anything that is available to anyone else is also by that very fact available to you; you only need to choose it.

Good choices open the door to health and happiness. What I mean by good choice is whatever works for you that you can or could share with those around you without a problem.

I have a friend who has a little pug-nosed dog who was born with two deformed front legs that are pretty much useless to him, as far as walking is concerned; so he moves around by sliding on his front legs and pushing with his back legs. When he wants to play or have fun with the other dogs or people he gets up on his back legs and dances around and plays as much as he wants to. He has become very skilled at this; in fact if you see him with all of the life and energy that he has, you would probably realize that he is not missing out on anything.

The point is that he doesn't know that this is supposed to be a handicap for him, so he just keep doing what he wants with what he's got and making life work for him.

He has not been told or conditioned into thinking that he is different and not like the other so-called normal dogs, so he just gets on with life.

I think that the main contributing factor is that when he gets up on his hind legs and starts to move like a dancer he gets a lot of attention; this is a treat or reward to him, so he keeps on.

This is what is often missing from people—they don't get enough praise or motivation in their lives, not enough treats. Most of the reason is that they wait for the world around them to do it. The problem is that this can or cannot happen, or happens not enough from others, so you have to take the responsibility for doing it for yourself.

Start and continue until it becomes habit (thirty days).

Remember the treats or rewards do not have to be big or extravagant; it can be as simple as a cup of coffee from your favorite place or dinner at your favorite restaurant, a piece of jewelry, dress, or pair of slacks that you really want—there are many ways to treat or reward yourself for achievements in your life, so treat yourself often, and this will become grand motivation towards health and happiness.

HAPPINESS

REQUIRES THAT YOU

KEEP LOOKING UNTIL YOU FIND

WHAT YOU ARE LOOKING FOR,

THEN YOU WILL BEGIN

TO LOOK FOR WHAT YOU FIND.

SIMPLE MEANS

SIMPLE HEALTH AND HAPPINESS

Health and happiness, like anything else in this life, has a price tag; in other words, you *gotta* pay for what you get—the payment eventually consists of decision and faith.

The decision is like going to the store and placing an order. You are saying, "This is what I want," or "This is what I would like to have." Once you place the order, faith becomes the vehicle carrying you towards your destination.

This is the point where God and the universe step in behind you to guide you on your chosen path towards health and happiness.

At this point you reach the conclusion that there are people in this life who enjoy health and happiness, and there are those who don't, and if there is anyone in this life enjoying health and happiness, that's proof that it's available, and if it is available, then it is also available to you; you simply have to choose it.

This is when you begin to create what you want from what is—the place where seeing is believing and believing is seeing.

So no matter where you are or who you are or what you are doing, you are able to see what you want in the situation. If you make a choice to see what you want in the situation, you at that point begin to not see or to tune out that which you do not want, so it fades further into the background until it eventually disappears from your life, and that which you have chosen to focus on becomes the whole picture.

Sure, you keep living and doing what you need to do to keep the day going, but now you put your wants and desires on the front burner and you keep your attention on them until they become all that you can see, and in the process you simply become.

THE AVERAGE PERSON

WILL FEEL BETTER AND ACCOMPLISH

MORE FROM A PAT ON THE BACK

THAN FROM A LITTLE MORE MONEY.

SIMPLE THOUGHT

I recently read that we have in the neighborhood of forty thousand thoughts a day, and that a big percentage of these thoughts are negative, and that negative thought seem to fly through the mind faster than positive thoughts—thoughts like "I don't like this" or "I don't like that," or "What if this does not work," or "What if I don't say the right thing," or "I don't like this person," or "What if someone doesn't like me," or "I will not get what I want," or "It's useless to ask, I won't get it anyway," or "It's a bad world," or "It's a bad life," and so on.

Is this true? Take a minute and ask yourself seriously, "Is this true?"

I think what we have to realize is that our health, happiness, and state of life are coming from these thoughts, because it's your programming. It's like people say about eating: "Garbage in, garbage out." Basically, it is like all of the information that you put into a computer from the day you buy it. If it is not something that is useful or that that can advance your life and purpose, then it can only take up space, slow down your computer, and become the source of many unneeded problems.

That is, until you decide to go back into your computer and delete each and every thing that is not serving your purpose. Your mind, unlike the computer, will have picked up things from other people and stored them, and because you are not always attentive to your thoughts (so as to change them to what you want them to be), these thoughts from other people bounce in, out, and around your mind, causing problems like stress, anxiety, insecurity, and unhappiness. This can take you to an unhealthy and unhappy existence.

To first just become conscious of your thoughts gives you the power to change or correct them, to disconnect from those that don't serve you and to connect to the ones that do serve you.

This is the place where you take control of your thinking and your life; this is the place where you decide to be healthy and happy.

So ask yourself, "Am I healthy? Am I living the life I like to live?" If you don't get a real yes, then it's time to go to the source of your life, your thinking.

You need to understand that if you have bad thoughts about yourself, your life, or anything in your life, even before you say or do anything, that bad thought will make you feel bad first.

This can be true unless you are always consciously making a choice, even with your thinking, and that choice can be to live, to be happy, to be healthy, and to have the best that this life has for you.

You start using that power of choice when you become conscious and start to move your thoughts to a better place.

There is a good side and a bad side to anything and everything. That is the foundation of freedom of choice—without things to choose between, there is no choice.

To become conscious shines light on the choices you have in your life. You then make the decision about what you want, or simply focus on the good and anything else will go away on its own.

Happy and healthy living is a choice—make this choice a habit and don't look back.

THOSE THINGS IN LIFE WORTH HAVING, ARE THOSE THINGS IN LIFE WORTH ASKING FOR

SIMPLE QUESTION

What is life? The opportunity

Why do we need life? We have chosen it

Do I have the power to change life? You can and you do, because every time you just breathe the entire universe must adjust (or change) to you, so the world around you must change from everything you do.

Can I fail? It is not possible within the context of a perfect universe where success is the only possibility, failure is a choice seen rather than a reality had.

Why are we here? Simply by choice to do what we do, just as every actor in a movie must play their part so that we can grasp and enjoy the whole of it, we must all play out our parts with great expectation that the movie of life will be a success.

Where does bad come from? Intention

Where does good come from? Intention

Where does life come from? Intention

Where does death come from? Intention

Where does joy and happiness come from? Intention

Where does unhappiness come from? Intention

Is there purpose? Yes, Creation, we create and recreate, from what was created, with intention this is purpose.

Why can't I have everything the way that I want it? *Un-intention* (it does not matter what is there if you are choosing not to see it).

Who is God? Everything

What is love? Everything else, and everything needed to apply

What do we need? Nothing, you have everything

What do we want? Everything

What is after death? Life

What is after life? Death

Where do we go then? Nowhere, you already are, only then you will know that you are there.

What is reality? What is and isn't.

How can I be true to myself? By accepting oneness with everyone else.

What is important in life? What you have chosen and what you are now doing, it is the only place, the chosen point in infinity.

Can I change the world? Yes, with a sincere thought.

Can I be a victim? If you believe you can.

Is life and all of this really necessary? Only as necessary as you need it to be.

Why is there pain in life? To help you see and recognize the flaw in you: creation.

Did Jesus exist? No

Did Jesus not exist? No

Which is true? Both depending on your belief.

What are miracles? Faith without end in solid form.

What are disasters? Like all other things, consciousness in motion.

Why can't I love everyone? You do and when you have gathered yourself unto yourself you will understand how it looks.

Romantic love? Romantic love is self recognition in its highest degree in physical form, just as we dislike in others what we dislike in ourselves most, we also love in others what we love most in ourselves.

Is peace possible? Yes, when you have learned to fear no part of yourself you will live in peace.

Can I solve the problems of the world? Yes, by solving your problems with the world.

When does life begin? It doesn't because it doesn't end, life is only matter changing form and taking on consciousness.

Is abortion wrong? It depends on who is judging and their perception.

Does God get angry? No, if you had total control over everything what would you need to get angry about.

What is mental illness? Illusion of an illusion not accepted

Did Jesus ever get frustrated or angry because it seemed like so many people were not doing what was right?

He didn't need to, he wasn't judging.

Is this really a perfect world? Could God have made anything imperfect?

Why don't others love me? They do, and when you allow yourself to feel love coming from yourself, you will also feel it from others.

Why do I feel lonely at times? We tend to associate loneliness with being alone, first if you believe in God you know that you are never alone, second just as the absence of sickness does not necessarily mean the presence of health the absence of people does not have to mean loneliness, just as sleep allows you to rejuvenate yourself physically, the absence of people can also be a time of mental rejuvenation, for even better relationships with people.

Is it possible to feel lonely in the presence of others? Yes, if for some reason you have chosen to mentally detach yourself, then you could feel lonely anytime.

Sometimes I feel that God has burdened me with so much with what I should do to try and make life right that I don't feel that I really have time to enjoy life beyond that, why? If you cannot find joy in your work it is neither God's work nor yours, it is more that you have for some reason chosen to burden yourself and are blaming God, as with "love thy neighbor as thyself", also "enjoy thy neighbor as thyself"; anything in your life that you cannot find time to enjoy is useless to you.

How do you know everything? We all do.

Why are you giving answers? Because I can.

Are they true? You decide.

"BE CAREFUL OF WHAT YOU ASK FOR,

YOU JUST MIGHT GET IT"

SIMPLE BELIEVING

I will see what I believe, I will hear what I believe, I will believe what I believe. When I believe what I believe, any and all justifications come in the choice that I have made. People have lived grand and glorious lives from what they believed; people have actually died from what they chose to believe. What is quite real to everyone else will simply become an illusion to me, if I choose to believe that it is.

"Faith can move mountains" or "Whosoever believeth shall not perish" finds its foundation in your choice to believe. If I choose to believe in love I will find all reasons and see all means to justify that choice that I have made, and it would be simply the same if I chose not to believe in love.

The best evidence of good and bad, sickness and health or disease, life and death lies in a place of which scientists have given us proof by not being able to put their finger on the cause. That place is the part that our belief system plays in every situation, simply because it cannot be measured by yards, meters, sight, sound, taste, smell, nor feel, so it becomes a long and empty pause on the tape recorder of scientists.

And where scientists have failed, faith has found its greatest foundation, within the confines of our belief system.

We do what we do because we have found reason and cause (and often in the scheme of overall life and health or well-being it can even be unjustifiable, logically speaking), while simply avoiding to look at anything outside of that in which we believe. The why of it can sometimes become the work of life that seems not so easy, for that is the very place where many are lost, lost in the belief that others have chosen through the illusion of their life, and often (as a magician does) seemingly justify all without question, until questioned. This is the place where laziness succumbs to belief (the beliefs of others, unquestioned).

I will be the witness of my Belief, by in effect questioning a grain of sand until it becomes a pearl, and perhaps what is too vast for my knowingness will in itself become the very proof of what I know.

I only need to smell the air, to see the sunrise, to see a baby to understand the endlessness and unboundedness of the universe, and to know that what or who is beyond this is its architect and builder.

When I find this place in myself and know it, I will find the who or what that is playing the strings on the instrument of my belief system. That is what I believe now.

GIVE YOUR THINKING ONLY TO THAT

WHICH SERVES YOU

AND YOUR HEALTH AND HAPPINESS,

AND IN THE PROCESS YOU SERVE GOD

AND ALL AROUND YOU FROM THAT

YOU HAVE.

TIH SIMPLE STATEMENT TO LIFE

You are my brother, my sister, my friend, no matter who you are, what you are, or where you are in the world, or in life—this is about you, me, and us.

What I owe to me, to you, and mostly to our creator is to find, to understand, and to share the best that he offers us, then I can rest from my work and live in oneness with all there in the highest place.

I have no reason to oppose, to fight, or to condemn anyone. It is he who stands as my strongest opposer, who stands to become my strongest ally, either through death (and we learn of what not to do) or through conversion, where he will bring forth the fullness of his opposition to encouragement. Only give to the creator and created that which rightfully belongs to them; that is the opportunity to live and rejoice in the life.

This statement that I cannot speak statistically on, but I can speak observantly on, is that failing health and disease are the top killers in this world along with starvation. Why? Mainly because our capitalist system teaches us that what you actually get out of a situation is more important than what you put into it. So if you look for the most prosperous industries in the world, I am guessing that you would find the food industry (yes it has been made into an industry), the pharmaceutical (medicine) industry, and the petroleum industry all at or near the top.

This does not mean that these people are my enemies; it simply means that the uninformed and the unconscious are leading us down a road to sickness, illness, and death, while instead of opening our eyes to see we blindly follow.

If we are to survive and live, we must not look to place blame for our lives with anyone else but ourselves ("I have found the enemy and the enemy is within"). Or, it is simply by my own hands that I will do more bad or more good in this life than anyone else will ever have the power to do.

"Seek ye the kingdom of heaven from within" is more about life here and now than anything else. It is about what we eat, drink, think, feel, live, breathe, and do, so that we rejoice in the space that God has given us to do that.

I must stress again that the full responsibility for this is only mine, because the truth is that we suffer not nearly as much from what others do to us as we do from what we do to ourselves.

There is no doubt in my mind that you are a special person put here in this life for a special reason, and your having this understanding allows you to see the truth of your existence, and to see in purpose a means to an end, which takes in account everything you do with yourself and others, so that at some point you become to identify as self.

So when we take full responsibility for ourselves we not only seek to live, but we live (from what we eat drink and think) our created purpose, with the end result being love, health, and happiness for me and all that I am.

I asked myself a question that got me to thinking: "Would I invite myself, my children, my family, and friends, or the people I care about to have a meal (food is one of the chief points of socialization in our lives), and then proceed to put a dead carcass (meat) on the plate, and around that some ground-up cardboard with motor oil, and sprinkle it with a sweet white poisonous chemical to make it look and taste good, and then dress all of this up to look like a royal wedding—could I or would I offer this to anyone that I care about and call it socialization?

Of course not, and you probably would not either, intentionally (this is pretty much what we consume and call food). So my question for you is: are you doing it unintentionally? That is the gist of what this book and system is about. Life is about what your intentions are for it, and that is life, love, and with love, health and happiness.

Our one goal with TIH is to assist you in your goal to health and happiness—and don't look back.

WHEN YOU COME TO A REAL

UNDERSTANDING ABOUT

WHAT YOU BELIEVE, YOU WILL KNOW

EXACTLY HOW, WHO, AND WHERE,

YOU ARE IN LIFE.

SIMPLE I

Where is the generation lost? If there is a generation lost then we are that generation, because we are the only generation.

Can we be lost? Yes we can, but not in a sense of a place that we can see or look for externally, but lost to ourselves. It is this place that we must seek, and not age, nor time, nor place, nor gender, nor perception must stand in the way of that. Why? Because it is where I find myself that I also find my life and the life that I am creating, and in turn that life that I see—it is truly with me that this all begins and ends.

It is in my purpose to find out who I am and in turn I find out who you are, and in my purpose to find out why I am here I can find out why you are here, and ultimately in my purpose to heal myself physically and mentally, I can also see how others can be healed. In my purpose to find peace in myself, I find peace in others; in my purpose to find worth in myself, I find worth in others; in my purpose to find reason in others, I find reason in myself; and ultimately in my purpose to find love in myself, I find love in others.

"Know thyself," "be truthful to thyn own self," "seek ye the kingdom of heaven from within," "hide not thy talents nor bury them in the earth below. As I have given to you display unto the world so that all, every man woman or child who sees you, will be inspired to do so," and "walk in the light of who you are and who they are, and what you are to become." Is it a matter of age? I ask, if you are ninety-two and you find yourself in the light of who you are, and you only live another day, you will have found your lifetime in happiness lived in that one day. It is true that this world has no trouble that I cannot find within myself, and as in sickness or in health, wherein lies the sickness also lies the means for the cure.

It is always the time that you find yourself and let the children of the world see you in the light of who you really are, and what you are here for, serving up your talents and truly "becoming the person that you would like to see in life." You cannot fail at becoming yourself and finding yourself, because you are always there and waiting to be found. You are here simply because the universe needs you here, but the universe cannot take from you what you do not choose to freely give, and that is the gift of who you are and the purpose you bring to life.

The children of Israel were lost in the desert of their soul, until they found purpose in themselves through a meaningful God who could be found in everything, and that was and is the miracle the miracle of who you are.

Serve yourself diligently unto the world, and all things to include happiness and love will be at your doorstep.

In love from love comes love.

THE REALIZATION OF THE ONENESS IS

THE ONLY CHANCE WE HAVE TO

SURVIVE THE REALITY OF IT ALL.

SIMPLE HEAVEN

It doesn't matter where you are if you are thinking is right. In fact, where you are is a result of some past thinking.

Some of our greatest saints have been subject to what we would consider to be some of the most horrific conditions, and at these moments they have experienced the height of Enlightenment and Joy. Why? Because right thought brings about right action.

It doesn't matter who you are, where you are, or what you do, it is all driven by your God-given ability to think, and in the seed of thought lies your God-power to create everything that your life is and will be about from this point on.

By the very nature of what God is, he cannot turn his back on anyone, nor will he abandon his creation. The creator by his nature has placed the love of his creation beyond the will of himself to take it away.

So the gates of Heaven are always open, and the only thing that can stand between you and God (Heaven) is your Thought, or your free will, which must be inaugurated by a thought.

You may be in the midst of a hurricane or flood, an earthquake, a relationship or job problem, in anger or depression – God summons you to Heaven through your thoughts, as it is sometimes in the deepest and darkest cave where we find gold. Quite often we only need walk over the hill that is in front of us to find Paradise, lying there in our path. Yes, any and all of Life's possibilities lie in front of you, directly behind your thought and belief.

The right Thought allows you to see God (the Good) in any situation. Essentially, we find what we look for. This can be God, Heaven, Love, Peace, Happiness, and so on, or all of these.

Yes, we are all unique individuals with our so-called problems seeming that way, but time and time again I have witnessed the Truth of the words of a Chinese Martial Arts Master, "There is no problem. The problem is You". If you take the You out of a problem, it ceases to exist.

The right thought is to find God in every situation, and the gates of Heaven will open to you. In that moment you will see, and every Thought becomes a step on the stairway to Heaven.

Sometimes we are too busy trying to be what we were yesterday to become what we are today, a New.

YOU CANNOT FAIL AT BECOMING

YOURSELF OR FINDING YOURSELF,

BECAUSE YOU ARE ALWAYS THERE

WAITING TO BE FOUND.

SIMPLE FAITH

Faith is the foundation and the chief motivating factor of life. It ties us to purpose and allows us to set, see, and walk towards our goals in life, instead of aimlessly wandering. It fills us with hope and dreams, and in the end, fulfillment.

I travel the world entertaining, seeking understanding of myself and my brothers and sisters here.

These are some of the simple understandings that I have come to around life.

I traveled for a time by myself but I was never alone, because the presence of God is always with me. This helped me to know that no matter where I was, or what was around me, or what I had to deal with, I always came out in a good place because I always had a good foundation to stand on, a foundation that is bigger, wiser, and stronger, with more ways and means than anything that I could encounter here on earth.

I have been always able to go forward in faith, and not look back.

During the process, I have noticed from talking with people (one of my life goals is to help people to live and love better) that they run into problems in and with their lives, in the way of unhappiness, insecurity, frustration, and depression, without any means of dealing with it all.

My counseling for people is very simple. First ask yourself, "If I am real and living here, then how could this be possible? Then ask yourself if it is possible that all of your body and its intimate and super-intelligent workings, along with the earth and all of what it produces in all of its perfection, and the entire universe as we can see seems to know how and what it should do to maintain and advance life and its own existence.

The question is, does your logical thinking tell you that this could all happen by chance? Now you are in the position to begin your search for life, your search to find God. When you find God, you find your reason, and it comes with a foundation that can withstand anything and everything that the world around you can throw at you.

We are born into a space, and we occupy that space while we are here. It is ours, and no one can take it. It is our choice what we choose to fill it with. We should know that most if not all of our problems in life are a result of fear, but fear and faith cannot occupy the same space. God or faith has to be a choice that you make.

Anything that will ever benefit you in life will require some effort on your part. As a popular song says, *"Nothin' from nothin' leaves nothin'.*
"You gotta have somethin'."

ANY AND ALL OF LIFE'S POSSIBILITIES

LIE IN FRONT OF YOU, DIRECTLY

BEHIND YOUR THOUGHTS AND

BELIEF.

WERE IT MY LAST WISH

WERE IT MY LAST WISH

I WOULD TEACH THE WORLD TO SMILE,

THEN I WOULD SMILE WITH THEM,

THEN I WOULD TEACH THE WORLD TO LAUGH,

THEN I WOULD LAUGH WITH THEM,

THEN I WOULD TEACH THE WORLD TO DANCE,

THEN I WOULD DANCE WITH THEM,

THEN I WOULD TEACH THE WORLD TO BELIEVE,

THEN I WOULD BELIEVE WITH THEM,

THEN I WOULD TEACH THE WORLD TO BE,

THEN I WOULD BE WITH THEM,

AND MOST OF ALL I WOULD TEACH THE WORLD TO LOVE,

THEN I WOULD LOVE WITH THEM.

LIFE IS A SIMPLE SITUATION WHERE

YOU CAN BEGIN WITH SOMETHING

AND, DEPENDING ON YOUR BELIEF,

END WITH EVERYTHING.

THE POSSIBILITIES ARE ALL WITH

YOU.

FINALE

WHO DO YOU THINK YOU ARE

You are God's creation at the point of perfection. You are grand in all of your own ways. You are only one step below the creator and endowed with the power of creation here, sent here with the power to engage through faith with your will. The universe bows to you and your wants. Why? Because you are empowered by the creator to create, so look at where you are, what you feel, how you live, and what you have—yes, look at it all and understand that it is all your own creation. Yes, God gave you the key to the room that is full of all the life you could want or need.

So how do you create? You create with every thought, and every wish, because every desire that you have must find its way into existence, and in this sense you are the only bidder at the auction of life, bidding on your own behalf.

You can awaken yourself to this reality at any time, because life awaits your command, so why not let this be the day that you wake up this moment and start living in health and happiness, because one more moment is too long to wait to start experiencing the grand dance of life.

This is your time to let go and let God, to turn your mind, turn your eyes, towards that which serves you and the universe totally through you, think only the thoughts, dream the dream, and put all else behind you. Then allow your faith to lead you; ask for and expect life on your terms. It is your time to really live a conscious life of happiness. It is your time to really live, love, be happy and prosperous.

It is a new day and a new life for someone so special … You.

HAPPY NEW LIFE.

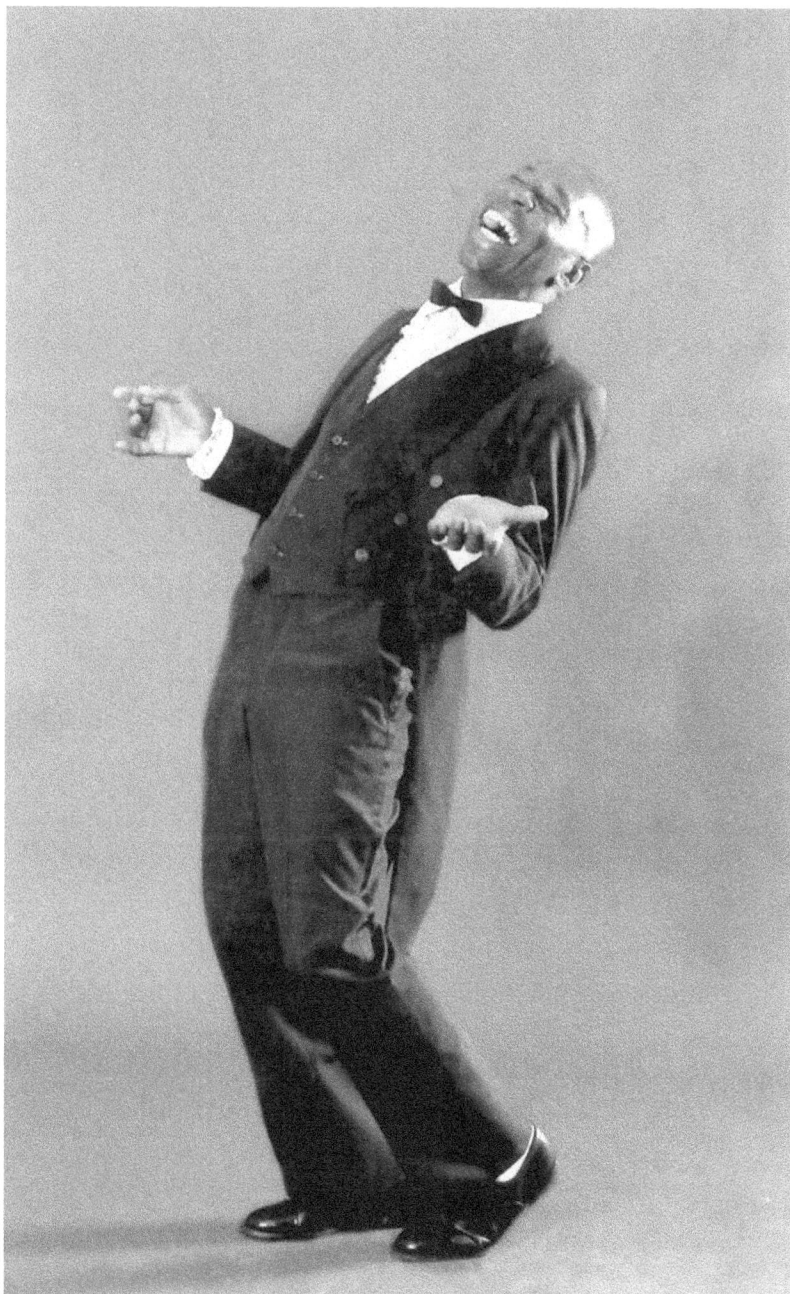

MOVIN' MELVIN BROWN

ALSO AVAILABLE BY THE AUTHOR

MUSIC CDS:

All of Me / Just for Fun / Let's Talk About Love /

A Man, A Magic, A Music / Just a little Country / Another Tyme /

Love on My Mind

Me, Ray Charles and Sammy Davis Jr / The Magic of You /

Soul to Soul (I Have a Dream) / Blues Country /

The Ray Charles Experience

Love Stormy Weather (single)

TIH Dance – Movin' with Melvin (2)

VIDEOS:

The Best of Movin' Melvin

TIH (Tap Into Health)

BOOKS:

As A Man Thinketh

Ordering information at *www.movinmelvin.com*

www.ingramcontent.com/pod-product-compliance
Lightning Source LLC
Chambersburg PA
CBHW052217270326
41931CB00011B/2388